DE-ESCALATING VIOLENCE IN HEALTHCARE

STRATEGIES TO REDUCE EMOTIONAL TENSION AND AGGRESSION

S. E. McKnight, DNP, MSN, BA, RN-BC

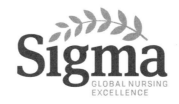

Sigma
GLOBAL NURSING
EXCELLENCE

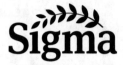

The Sigma Theta Tau International Honor Society of Nursing (Sigma) is a nonprofit organization whose mission is advancing world health and celebrating nursing excellence in scholarship, leadership, and service. Founded in 1922, Sigma has more than 135,000 active members in over 90 countries and territories. Members include practicing nurses, instructors, researchers, policymakers, entrepreneurs, and others. Sigma's more than 530 chapters are located at more than 700 institutions of higher education throughout Armenia, Australia, Botswana, Brazil, Canada, Colombia, England, Ghana, Hong Kong, Japan, Jordan, Kenya, Lebanon, Malawi, Mexico, the Netherlands, Nigeria, Pakistan, Philippines, Portugal, Puerto Rico, Singapore, South Africa, South Korea, Swaziland, Sweden, Taiwan, Tanzania, Thailand, the United States, and Wales. Learn more at www.sigmanursing.org.

Sigma Theta Tau International
550 West North Street
Indianapolis, IN, USA 46202

To order additional books, buy in bulk, or order for corporate use, contact Sigma Marketplace at 888.654.4968 (US/Canada toll-free) or +1.317.634.8171 (International).

To request a review copy for course adoption, email solutions@sigmamarketplace.org or call 888.654.4968 (US/Canada toll-free) or +1.317.634.8171 (International).

To request author information, or for speaker or other media requests, contact Sigma Marketing at 888.634.7575 (US/Canada toll-free) or +1.317.634.8171 (International).

ISBN: 9781948057493
EPUB ISBN: 9781948057509
PDF ISBN: 9781948057516
MOBI ISBN: 9781948057523

Library of Congress Cataloging-in-Publication data

Names: McKnight, S. E., 1954- author. | Sigma Theta Tau International, issuing body.
Title: De-escalating violence in healthcare : strategies to reduce emotional tension and
   aggression / S. E. McKnight.
Description: First. | Indianapolis, IN : Sigma Theta Tau International
   Honor Society of Nursing, [2020] | Includes bibliographical references. | Summary: "This
   book is a comprehensive guidebook of therapeutic de-escalation techniques for nurses and other
   healthcare professionals to improve safety in healthcare facilities. Readers will explore the concepts
   of aggression (including risk factors), de-escalation, and therapeutic communication. They
   will also learn how to perform mental status assessments, manage and even prevent aggressive
   behavior, and practice conflict resolution, and--when faced with individuals with depressive
   disorders, suicidal ideation, and/or self-injurious behavior--engage in crisis intervention.
   Specific therapeutic interventions for difficult behavioral issues associated with schizophrenia,
   dementia, bipolar disorder, cognitive impairment, anxiety and panic disorders are also covered,
   as are stress-management techniques to help patients cope, tips for creating a caring and healing
   environment to stop violence before it starts, and a framework for building a healthcare violence
   prevention program. Nursing students and healthcare professionals of all educational levels will
   find this book to be immensely valuable. De-escalation is one of the most valuable skills a healthcare
   worker can possess. Indeed, all healthcare workers need this vital skill to help ensure their safety in
   the healthcare environment. It's not uncommon for healthcare professionals to encounter an agitated
   or aggressive person. How that healthcare worker responds will dictate whether the situation is
   defused or escalated--perhaps even resulting in physical violence. The goal of this book is to ensure
   the result is the former--to prevent healthcare violence, and to foster a safe healthcare workplace that
   benefits all and promotes peace and safety for everyone"-- Provided by publisher.
Identifiers: LCCN 2019021730 | ISBN 9781948057493 | ISBN 9781948057523 (mobi) |
   ISBN 9781948057516 (pdf) | ISBN 9781948057509 (epub)
Subjects: MESH: Workplace Violence--prevention & control | Health Facilities |
   Aggression--psychology | Crisis Intervention | Health Personnel | Nurses Instruction
Classification: LCC RA969.9 | NLM WX 185 | DDC 362.11028/9--dc23
LC record available at https://lccn.loc.gov/2019021730

First Printing, 2019

Publisher: Dustin Sullivan
Acquisitions Editor: Emily Hatch
Development Editor: Kate Shoup
Cover Designer: Rebecca Batchelor
Interior Design/Page Layout: Kim Scott/Bumpy Design
Illustrator: Michael Tanamachi

Managing Editor: Carla Hall
Project Editor: Kate Shoup
Publications Specialist: Todd Lothery
Copy Editor: Erin Geile
Proofreader: Gill Editorial Services
Indexer: Larry Sweazy

DEDICATION

This book is dedicated to the cause of peace and to all those who advocate for peace and nonviolence. They are the living instruments of true peace!

ACKNOWLEDGMENTS

I would like to acknowledge the editors and staff of Sigma Theta Tau International Honor Society of Nursing for their dedication to education and safety and for making this book possible to promote the cause of violence prevention and peace.

ABOUT THE AUTHOR

S. E. McKnight, DNP, MSN, BA, RN-BC, is a career mental health educator who has served in a compassionate mental health nursing practice for more than 22 years. Her specialty is de-escalation training to prevent violence and promote holistic wellness and recovery. No longer a skill practiced only by the mental health disciplines, de-escalation has become a critical skill for all healthcare practices, domains, and disciplines. McKnight has had the privilege of witnessing the dramatic transformation of chaotic healthcare environments into safe, caring, and healing environments with the implementation of de-escalation education programs for all healthcare staff. Presently McKnight teaches mental health nursing at the University of West Florida in Pensacola, Florida, where she educates the next generation of healthcare professionals in safe, holistic nursing care.

She completed a doctor of nursing practice with honors from the University of Alabama and received both her master of nursing science and bachelor of art from the University of South Alabama. Prior to that, she received her associate in nursing from Bishop State Community College. She is a board-certified nursing educator in the field of mental health nursing practice, nursing professional development, and holistic nursing and has received numerous awards for academic excellence in mental health nursing education.

McKnight develops and publishes research in many academic scholarly journals and has contributed to several books. She developed the first competency-based mental health learning needs assessment for professional nursing practice. This needs assessment is published in the American Psychiatric Association database as a best practice instrument for use in both research and education. Her clinical experience has included psychiatric consultation and liaison nursing, addiction recovery counseling, psychiatric emergency department triage, and crisis counseling. McKnight has also worked as an educator for inpatient adult, geriatric, child, and adolescent behavioral health facilities. While working in various clinical positions, she developed and taught specialized evidence-based education programs focused on de-escalation and violence prevention. McKnight delivers workshops and seminars on violence prevention education programs focused on safety.

She is an active member of many professional nursing organizations, including the National League for Nursing, the American Psychiatric Nurses Association, the American Nurses Association, and the American Holistic Nurses Association. McKnight divides her time between clinical practice, training, consulting, scholarly writing, and research.

TABLE OF CONTENTS

About the Author vii
Introduction. xv

1 De-Escalation for Holistic Wellness 1
   The Three Interventional Pathways for Aggression 2
   Response Tools. 4
   The De-Escalation Process 5
   Assess the Situation 6
   Implement Safety Measures 7
   Apply De-Escalation Techniques 7
   After the Incident: Debriefing, Reporting, and Documenting 8
   Working With Family Members and Caregivers. 9
   References. 11

2 Variables and Risk Factors for Aggression 13
   Patient Variables 15
   Environmental Variables 16
   Caregiver Variables. 18
   Patient and Caregiver Interaction Variables 20
   Other Risk Factors. 20
   References. 25

3 Assessing an Escalating Situation for Early Intervention . . . 29
   The Aggression Continuum and the Escalation Cycle 30
   The Assault Cycle 34
   Triggers of Aggressive or Violent Behavior 36
   Escalating Behaviors. 39
   Assessing Patient Behavior for Signs of Agitation 41
   The Importance of Early Intervention. 42
   References. 42

4 De-Escalation Techniques **45**

Verbal Techniques for De-Escalation 46

Distraction for De-Escalation 48

Calming Comfort Measures 49

Reorienting the Patient to Reality............................... 50

De-Stress to De-Escalate 50

Milieu Management 51

Principles of Safe and Effective De-Escalation.................... 52

References.. 56

5 Therapeutic Communication for De-Escalation **59**

The Therapeutic Communication Cycle 60

Verbal and Nonverbal Communication 61

Communication Contexts....................................... 63

Criteria for Successful Communication........................... 64

Fundamental Elements of Therapeutic Communication 65

Therapeutic Communication Techniques.......................... 66

Tips to Establish Trust and Therapeutic Rapport.................. 69

References.. 71

6 Stress-Management Techniques. **75**

The Fundamental Elements of All Human Beings 76

The Stress Response... 78

Types of Stress 79

Common Causes of Stress in the Modern World................... 80

Holistic Stress Management 81

Diaphragmatic Breathing 83

Mental Imagery... 84

Meditation... 87

Progressive Muscular Relaxation 88

References.. 90

7 Conflict Resolution **93**

Benefits of Conflict Resolution 94

Types of Conflict.. 95

Conflict-Resolution Styles...................................... 95

Elements of Conflict Resolution 97

Rules for Open Communication 99

References.. 100

8 Crisis Intervention 103
   Stages of Crisis Development 104
   Common Crisis State Behaviors 105
   Types of Crises 106
   Three Phases of Crisis Intervention 107
   The Importance of Communication During a Crisis 109
   References 110

9 Managing Mental Health Emergencies 113
   Common Mental Health Emergencies 115
   Performing an Emergency Mental Health Assessment 116
   Aiding the Suicidal Patient 118
   Aiding the Patient Suffering From Alcohol or Substance Abuse 119
   Aiding the Violent Patient 121
   References 124

10 Performing a Mental Status Assessment 125
    Performing a Legal Status Assessment .128
    Assessing the Patient's Physical Appearance 128
    Evaluating Alertness, Orientation, Behavior, Attitude,
       Affect, and Mood 129
    Analyzing Thought Processes, Thought Content, Attention,
       Concentration, and Memory 132
    Appraising Judgment, Insight, and Intellect 134
    Noting Hallucinations and Delusions 134
    Assessing Speech and Motor Activity 135
    Additional Mental Status Assessments .137
    Performing a Risk Assessment 137
    Formulating a De-Escalation Plan 143
    References 146

11 De-Escalation of Patients With Mental Disorders 149
    Assessing and De-Escalating Patients With Schizophrenia 150
    Assessing and De-Escalating Patients With Bipolar Disorder 154
    Assessing and De-Escalating Patients With Major
       Depressive Disorder 157
    Assessing and De-Escalating Patients With Panic Disorder 159
    Comparing Conditions 163
    References 166

12 De-Escalation of Patients Exhibiting
    Non-Suicidal Self-Injury (NSSI) Behavior 169
    Origins of NSSI Behavior 171
    Assessing Patients With NSSI Behavior 173
    Preventing Escalation of Patients With NSSI Behavior 174
    De-Escalation Techniques for Patients With NSSI Behavior 175
    Differentiating NSSI Behavior From Suicidal Ideation 176
    References 177

13 De-Escalation of Patients With Dementia 181
    Assessing a Dementia Patient 182
    Preventing Escalation With Dementia Patients 184
    Effective De-Escalation Practices for Dementia Patients 187
    Maintaining Quality of Life for Dementia Patients 189
    References 190

14 De-Escalation of Patients With Delirium 193
    Origins of Delirium 195
    Assessing Patients With Delirium 195
    Preventing Escalation of Patients With Delirium 196
    De-Escalation Techniques for Patients With Delirium 198
    Working With Family Members 200
    Ensuring the Safety of Patients With Delirium 201
    References 201

15 De-Escalation of "Difficult" Patients 203
    Origins of Difficult Behaviors 205
    Assessing a Difficult Patient 206
    Preventing Escalation With Difficult Patients 207
    Effective De-Escalation Practices for Difficult Patients 208
    Aiding Difficult Patients Who Are Elderly 211
    References 212

16 De-Escalation of Angry Patients 213
    Types of Expressions of Anger 214
    Origins of Anger and Common Anger Triggers 216
    Assessing the Angry Patient 217
    Preventing Patients From Expressing Anger Inappropriately 218
    De-Escalation Techniques for Angry Patients 220
    References 222

17 Staying Safe During De-Escalation **223**

   Implement Door Safety Protocols. 224
   Pay Attention to Your Surroundings 225
   Give the Patient Room 225
   Watch Your Body Language 225
   Be Mindful of Hair and Accessories 227
   Don't Threaten the Patient 228
   Keep a Coworker Nearby 228
   References. 231

18 After the Incident **233**

   Debriefing With the Patient and Staff. 234
   Reporting and Documenting a De-Escalation Encounter 236
   References. 238

19 Creating a Calming, Caring, and Healing Healthcare
   Environment **239**

   Creating a Caring and Healing Physical Environment 240
   Fostering Caring and Healing Healthcare Environments Through
      Staff Interactions 241
   A Model for Caring Behavior 243
   Caring Theory 243
   References. 246

20 Developing a Healthcare Violence-Prevention Plan **247**

   Addressing Patient Factors. 248
   Addressing Environmental Factors. 251
   Addressing Caregiver Factors 255
   Putting It All Together. 258
   In Conclusion. 262
   References. 263

   Index 265

INTRODUCTION

In 2002, the World Health Organization recognized violence as a global health priority with significant health, social, and economic consequences. It's no wonder. Anger, aggression, and violence permeate every aspect of our culture—including healthcare organizations (Liss & McCaskell, 1994).

In a 2014 survey of registered nurses and nursing students, 21% of respondents reported being physically assaulted at work during a 12-month period, and more than 50% reported being verbally abused. Experts also estimate that fewer than half of all such incidents are actually reported (Occupational Safety and Health Administration [OSHA], 2015).

The same year, the Bureau of Labor Statistics reported that 52% of reported workplace violence incidents occurred in healthcare settings. Indeed, a violent incident is over four times more likely to occur in a healthcare setting than in any other professional workplace. As for injuries suffered by healthcare professionals at work, 80% of these are caused by patients (OSHA, 2015)—although healthcare workers must also contend with agitated family members of patients and stressed-out coworkers. Experts estimate that 50% of healthcare workers will encounter violence at least once in their healthcare careers (Findorff, McGovern, Wall, Gerberich, & Alexander, 2004).

The number of violent incidents in healthcare settings has continued to rise (The Joint Commission, 2018). There are various reasons for this. One is that our chaotic modern world fosters considerable stress and conflict, which naturally seeps into the healthcare environment. Here are several other reasons:

- A lack of organizational policies regarding de-escalation

- A lack of training of healthcare staff in de-escalation

- The stressful environments of many medical facilities (due to crowding, long waits, receiving bad news, and so on)

- Increased gang activity and crime that invade the healthcare workplace with the traumatic results of violence

- Increased alcohol and substance use or addiction (The Joint Commission, 2018)

- Large numbers of domestic disputes among patients and visitors

- The increasing presence of firearms and weapons brought into healthcare facilities by patients and visitors

- Inadequate security at healthcare facilities

- A lack of availability of mental health personnel to resolve conflicts that arise

- Frequent understaffing of healthcare facilities (meaning fewer available staff to provide care and safety)

- Healthcare facilities in which staff work in isolation

- Healthcare facilities in which staff can be easily trapped by an aggressive patient or other party

- Poor lighting in corridors, rooms, and parking lots that allow for easy assault

- Healthcare facilities that lack emergency communication tools such as cellphones or call bells to obtain emergency assistance

- Unrestricted public access to hospitals and clinics allowing for the entry of criminal elements

There is also a shortage of community mental health centers—leaving traditional medical facilities to provide access to these services. The de-institutionalization of the mentally ill has caused large numbers of the chronically mentally ill to enter the mainstream community without access to adequate mental healthcare.

All this has taken a growing financial and human toll on the nation's 15 million healthcare workers and on the hospitals, long-term care centers, and other facilities that employ them. Too many healthcare professionals feel unsafe at work. Indeed, this lack of safety has driven many nurses and other healthcare professionals to leave the industry entirely (The Joint Commission, 2018). Often nurses stay in nursing for about as long as it took them to obtain their professional education before leaving nursing permanently (Blegen, Spector, Lynn, Barnsteiner, & Ulrich, 2017).

This has the unfortunate effect of adding to the existing nurse shortage; and, as nurse-to-patient ratios fall, the risk of violence continues to increase, and the cycle continues.

The growing problem of violence in the healthcare setting has prompted many healthcare executives, providers, and policymakers to take action in myriad ways. Unfortunately, these efforts have proven largely ineffective, insofar as the number of violent incidents has yet to decrease. That means nurses and other front-line providers must identify effective tactics and tools to handle aggressive patients (and others).

The first and most beneficial technique to prevent healthcare violence is de-escalation training. *De-escalation* is the process of helping others regain self-control by using therapeutic communication and interventions to lower the emotional tension. De-escalation is a nonpharmacological approach for preventing violence—in healthcare facilities and anywhere else. Safety begins with assessment and early intervention with effective violence prevention tools (OSHA, 2016).

Research shows that when a situation involving an aggressive person is effectively de-escalated, violence is reduced. De-escalation can also help healthcare facilities avoid containment (takedown) episodes, which can lead to patient and staff injuries, as well as avoid using tranquilizers, restraints, or seclusion to ensure the safety of agitated patients and those around them. De-escalation is the least restrictive intervention recommended by the Joint Commission on Accreditation (2018) to prevent aggression/violence. It also decreases patient stress and anxiety and allows agitated patients to feel understood. De-escalation as a first response is key to reducing violent incidents in healthcare facilities.

De-escalation doesn't just happen. Training in de-escalation techniques is essential. That's where this book comes in. It serves as a comprehensive guidebook of therapeutic de-escalation techniques for nurses and other healthcare professionals to improve safety in healthcare facilities.

Readers will explore the concepts of aggression (including risk factors), de-escalation, and therapeutic communication. They will also learn how to perform mental status assessments, manage and even prevent aggressive behavior, practice conflict resolution, and—when faced with individuals with depressive disorders, suicidal ideation, or self-injurious behavior—engage in crisis intervention. Specific therapeutic interventions for difficult behavioral issues associated with schizophrenia, dementia, bipolar disorder, cognitive impairment, anxiety, and panic disorders are also covered, as are stress-management techniques to help patients cope, tips for creating a caring and healing environment to stop violence before it starts, and a framework for building a healthcare violence prevention program. Nursing students and healthcare professionals of all educational levels will find this book to be immensely valuable.

De-escalation is one of the most valuable skills a healthcare worker can possess. Indeed, all healthcare workers need this vital skill to help ensure their safety in the healthcare environment. It's not uncommon for healthcare professionals to encounter an agitated or aggressive person. How that healthcare worker responds will dictate whether the situation is defused or escalated—perhaps even resulting in physical violence. The goal of this book is to ensure the result is the former—to prevent healthcare violence, and to foster a safe healthcare workplace that benefits all and promotes peace and safety for everyone.

REFERENCES

Blegen, M. A., Spector, N., Lynn, M. R., Barnsteiner, J., & Ulrich, B. T. (2017). Newly licensed RN retention: Hospital and nurse characteristics. *The Journal of Nursing Administration, 47*(10), 508–514.

Findorff, M. J., McGovern, P. M., Wall, M., Gerberich, S. G., & Alexander, B. (2004). Risk factors for work related violence in a health care organization. *Injury Prevention, 10*(5), 296–302.

The Joint Commission. (2018, April 16). *Sentinel event alert 59: Physical and verbal violence against health care workers.* Retrieved from https://www.jointcommission.org/sea_issue_59/

Liss, G. M., & McCaskell, L. (1994). Violence in the workplace. *Canadian Medical Association Journal, 151*(9), 1243–1246.

Occupational Safety and Health Administration. (2015). *Workplace violence in healthcare.* Retrieved from https://www.osha.gov/publications/osha3826.pdf

Occupational Safety and Health Administration. (2016). *Guidelines for preventing workplace violence for healthcare and social service workers.* Retrieved from https://www.osha.gov/Publications/osha3148.pdf

1

DE-ESCALATION FOR HOLISTIC WELLNESS

"If we want to reap the harvest of peace and justice in the future, we will have to sow seeds of nonviolence, here and now, in the present."

–Mairead Corrigan Maguire

OBJECTIVES

- Identify the three interventional pathways for aggression

- Identify key response tools

- Find out the steps to de-escalation

- Describe the assessment phase

- Understand the importance of safety measures

- Identify de-escalation techniques

- Find out what to do after a de-escalation incident

- Consider how to work with family members and caregivers

At present, healthcare workers experience the highest rate of workplace violence injuries. During the past decade, approximately two-thirds of nonfatal injuries due to workplace violence involved healthcare workers (The National Institute for Occupational Safety and Health [NIOSH], n.d.).

De-escalation is a valuable tool in the prevention of workplace violence. *De-escalation* involves using therapeutic communication and interventions to defuse agitated patients to prevent them from escalating to dangerous levels of aggression or violence.

The focus of de-escalation is on prevention of violence. De-escalation techniques stop violence before it starts (American Psychiatric Association, American Psychiatric Nurses Association, & National Association of Psychiatric Health Systems, 2007). Early intervention with de-escalation techniques breaks the cycle of escalation, defuses the situation, and prevents patients from acting on their aggression in a violent manner.

De-escalation is a critical element of all workplace violence prevention programs. The NIOSH and The Joint Commission (JC) on Accreditation recommend training initiatives in de-escalation for all healthcare workers as an essential part of a workplace violence prevention program.

THE THREE INTERVENTIONAL PATHWAYS FOR AGGRESSION

So, what should you do when, after assessing the situation, you determine that you are in fact dealing with an aggressive patient? There are three interventional pathways for aggressive behavior (Chou, Kaas, & Richie, 1996). These pathways are as follows:

- **Psychological.** When faced with an agitated or aggressive patient, this is the first interventional pathway you should take. This pathway helps address symptoms, decrease distress and anxiety, and in many cases avert a negative outcome. With this pathway, the primary nursing intervention involves verbal de-escalation techniques—for example, encouraging the patient to express feelings to relieve the pressure. Other de-escalation techniques, such as distraction techniques, are also effective. For example, you might offer to turn on the television, offer the patient a book or magazine to read, or accompany the patient for a walk. Finally, you could encourage the person to perform relaxation exercises such as deep breathing.

Limit-setting is particularly important with this interventional pathway. And as always, the earlier the intervention, the more effective it will be.

> ✅ **NOTE** Using a psychological de-escalation approach as a first response is key to reducing episodes of aggression. This approach is the least restrictive intervention. It decreases distress and anxiety, increases the chances of the aggressive patient feeling understood, and in many cases helps to avert negative outcomes (Cowin et al., 2003).

- **Pharmacological.** If psychological de-escalation interventions fail and dangerous escalation persists, the second interventional pathway is the pharmacological pathway (Patel et al., 2018). This pathway involves administering sedatives, benzodiazepines, or short-acting barbiturates to calm the patient's aggressive behavior (Chou et al., 1996; Paton et al., 2018). If a medication is offered, it is a PRN (when needed) medication and not a chemical restraint. A PRN medication is a low-dose medication that calms agitated or aggressive patients but allows them to be responsive to verbal stimuli and their environment, and able to complete all normal activities of daily living such as feeding, bathing, and dressing. If it's clear that psychological de-escalation efforts are failing, it's best to advance to this interventional pathway sooner rather than later—before the patient loses control completely. Be aware that every person metabolizes medications at a different rate. When administering a PRN medication for agitation or aggression, it is therefore important to continue using verbal de-escalation techniques until the person calms down and regains self-control. The JC (2019) also requires documentation of de-escalation attempts prior to PRN medication administration as a best-practice quality measure. Finally, be sure to monitor the patient for any side effects.

> ⚠️ **CAUTION** A chemical restraint is an inappropriate use of a psychotropic medication to manage or control behavior, leaving the patient unresponsive or unable to complete activities of daily living (JC, 2019). Healthcare and medical facilities do not use chemical restraints.

- **Physical.** Physical interventions could include physical containment, such as seclusion or a therapeutic containment (takedown), show of support (when staff members gather to assist a colleague in danger when an emergency response code is issued), and use of restraints (applied and

monitored as per facility policy and with a physician/psychiatrist order).
Note that using physical restraints should be a last resort—done only when
the patient is an imminent danger to himself or to others and all other
interventions have failed. The JC (2019) requires nurses to document all
de-escalation interventions attempted prior to the application of a restraint
or seclusion. There are dangers and risks of re-traumatization associated
with use of restraints and takedowns. Mental health facilities have moved to
using one-to-one monitoring in a private room with an open doorway as a
safer and more humane alternative to the physical pathway.

With all three pathways, continuous monitoring must be performed until the
patient becomes stable and calm.

In addition to these interventional pathways, it may be necessary to implement
psychosocial interventions to de-escalate an agitated or aggressive individual
(Littrell & Littrell, 1998). This might include a visit from a social worker to
address housing, transportation, or other psychosocial issues that may be triggering the patient's negative behavior. This can greatly reduce the patient's stress
and therefore reduce the risk of violence.

> ☑ **NOTE** This book focuses primarily on psychological de-escalation
> techniques. The psychological pathway of de-escalation is the effective
> and noncoercive approach to managing aggressive behavior. De-escalation
> improves safety and in many instances reduces or even prevents the use of
> PRN medication and restraint or seclusion. The new paradigm for managing
> agitated behavior is engaging the patient, establishing a collaborative rela-
> tionship, and verbally de-escalating the patient (Richmond et al., 2012). When
> de-escalation is initiated with genuine commitment, successful outcomes that
> promote optimal well-being and safety can be achieved.

RESPONSE TOOLS

When faced with an aggressive patient, you have a few tools at your disposal to
help prevent escalation. All three of these tools are used in conjunction with the
psychological intervention pathway. The tools are as follows:

- **De-escalation.** This involves encouraging the agitated patient to verbalize the anger source. This often causes the anger to dissipate and helps
  the patient calm down. Chapter 4, "De-Escalation Techniques," discusses
  de-escalation techniques in more detail.

- **Conflict resolution.** This involves collaborating and negotiating between two conflicting parties until a resolution that is agreeable to both parties is achieved. Chapter 7, "Conflict Resolution," discusses this topic in more detail.

- **Problem-solving.** This involves helping the patient identify the problem, sharing information with the patient that pertains to the problem (if applicable), brainstorming possible solutions, and implementing the solution most likely to resolve the problem.

> **? TIP** During the problem-solving process, have patients write down whatever problem is troubling them and needs resolving, and the list of possible solutions developed during the brainstorming session. Then ask them to rank each solution in the list from 1 (best) to 10 (worst). The top-ranking solution is the one patients should enact. (If patients have more than one problem, have them write them all down, and solve each problem one at a time.)

> **? TIP** Consider performing a mental health learning needs assessment for staff to identify any gaps in de-escalation knowledge. If gaps exist, implement training programs to ensure all staff are up to speed.

THE DE-ESCALATION PROCESS

The de-escalation process involves five key steps:

1. Assess the situation.

2. Implement safety measures.

3. Apply de-escalation techniques.

4. Debrief.

5. Report and document the incident.

These phases are discussed in more detail in this chapter and throughout the book.

ASSESS THE SITUATION

Aggression occurs on a continuum. This continuum involves a trigger phase, an escalation phase, and a crisis phase. It is important to assess the situation at hand to identify where on the aggression continuum the patient is. In addition to an aggression continuum, there is an assault cycle. This cycle, articulated by Caplan (1970), has six phases: activation, escalation, crisis, recovery, post-crisis depression, and stabilization. This information is important during the assessment phase. When faced with an agitated patient, it's important to intervene as early in the aggression continuum and assault cycle as possible by applying de-escalation techniques to prevent escalation to harmful levels of agitation. The aggression continuum and assault cycle are discussed in more detail in Chapter 3, "Assessing an Escalating Situation for Early Intervention."

In addition to identifying where an agitated patient is on the aggression continuum and assault cycle, it's important to identify key types of risk factors. These include patient risk factors, environmental risk factors, and caregiver risk factors.

To identify patient risk factors, you should perform a mental status assessment upon admission. Mental status assessments are a standard operating practice at mental health facilities. Many medical health facilities have also begun incorporating mental status assessments into their practice for a holistic assessment focused on recovery and safety. This assessment involves identifying risk factors and triggers for escalation. This information helps healthcare staff implement violence prevention or intervention measures as needed. The assessment also entails identifying the patient's preferred methods of de-escalation. Finally, the assessment involves observing the patient's body language for clues of escalation, such as clenched fists or a tense posture. (This type of observation should be conducted even after admission for the duration of the patient's stay.) Chapter 10, "Performing a Mental Status Assessment," discusses this process in more detail.

Environmental risk factors should also be identified during the assessment phase. These might include overcrowding or excessive noise. If patients state that noise makes them agitated, then they should be moved to a quieter area of the unit.

Finally, caregiver risk factors should be recognized. Caregivers must be very self-aware to be effective in de-escalation. They must also have training in de-escalation techniques and exercise good self-control. Caregivers should assess whether they have these qualities and skills. If they do not, they should turn over the task of de-escalation to someone who does in the short term, and seek training in the long term. De-escalation is a team endeavor. The best person for effective de-escalation is the person who has training in de-escalation techniques; can retain self-control; and can maintain a calm, professional demeanor.

> ☑ **NOTE** Chapter 2, "Variables and Risk Factors for Aggression," discusses patient, environmental, and caregiver risk factors in more detail.

IMPLEMENT SAFETY MEASURES

Safety is a paramount concern in any de-escalation scenario. An important safety practice is to use the "buddy system" in any behavioral emergency. You might activate this using silent hand signals, calling in a code, or pressing a panic button. You should never attempt to de-escalate a patient alone. Chapter 17, "Staying Safe During De-Escalation," covers critical safety measures in more detail.

APPLY DE-ESCALATION TECHNIQUES

De-escalation techniques are effective in calming patients; reducing containment (takedowns), which can cause patient and staff injuries; and reducing the use of restraints and seclusion, which can retraumatize patients.

The de-escalation techniques you use should be specific to the nature and acuity of the event. Therapeutic communication—asking open-ended questions to encourage patients to verbalize their issues such as, "What are you feeling right now?" or, "How can I help you?"—is key. So is ensuring you give the agitated patient space, stand near a door or exit for safety, demonstrate a supportive stance with your palms up, and exhibit a calm and caring demeanor.

Five Principles of Aggression Prevention

Of course, it's better to prevent aggression than to manage it once it occurs. The following five principles of aggression prevention can help you achieve this:

- **Screen for aggression risk factors upon admission.** This will enable you to identify problem patients and potential issues early on (Owen, Tarantello, Jones, & Tennant, 1998; for more on screening for risk factors, see Chapter 10).

■ **Foster a healing treatment environment.** A calm environment can greatly reduce inpatient aggression.

■ **Be proactive.** Prepare in advance so you're ready in case of danger. Make sure your cellphone is with you, you've activated the "buddy system" for safety, and you're within sight of other staff for safety. (For more information, see Chapter 17.)

■ **Be alert and aware of your surroundings for safety.** Notice if there are weapons of opportunity that could be wielded against or thrown at you, such as a chair or lamp, within reach of the patient. If possible, remove these objects or move the patient away from them for safety.

■ **Use one-to-one monitoring for patients at risk of escalation.** One-to-one monitoring is when one nurse watches one patient for safety, giving the patient undivided attention. This interaction should be therapeutic rather than custodial in nature. The nurse should use therapeutic communication and de-escalation techniques to prevent escalation and violence while developing therapeutic rapport with the patient.

If prevention efforts fail, and a patient becomes agitated or aggressive, it's best to intervene right away.

? TIP The best de-escalation technique is to intervene at the first sign of aggression. Look for body language clues such as clenched fists or a tense posture.

AFTER THE INCIDENT: DEBRIEFING, REPORTING, AND DOCUMENTING

After an aggressive episode is over, when the patient is restored to a calm state and has regained self-control, there are three critical actions that must be taken.

One critical action is a debriefing. This should be conducted with everyone involved in the incident—including the patient. This debriefing involves seeking answers to a series of simple questions:

■ Who was involved?

■ What happened?

- Where did it happen?

- What caused it to happen?

- How can we prevent it from happening again?

Debriefing is a Joint Commission (JC) (2019) mandated process for all mental health facilities. In addition, all debriefings must occur within 24 hours of the incident. The results of the debriefing should be documented and made part of the electronic health record.

Debriefing should never be punitive. The point of any debriefing is to identify ways to prevent the same type of aggressive episode from happening again in the future. Debriefings also help those who experienced the event to process any trauma associated with it.

Another critical action is to report the incident to the provider on duty, such as the physician, psychiatrist, or nurse practitioner, as well as the nurse manager or supervisor on duty. Some facilities may also require an incident report be completed.

Finally, the incident must be documented. This verifies the use of best practice, least-restrictive de-escalation interventions, as required by the JC. Failure to document de-escalation attempts prior to using PRN medication, restraints, or seclusion may result in the facility being marked as substandard in care by the JC (Snorrason & Biering, 2018).

WORKING WITH FAMILY MEMBERS AND CAREGIVERS

Healthcare staff don't just deal with patients. They also must care for the patient's family. A *family* is defined as a group of two or more people living together related by bonds of blood, marriage, or adoption (Boyd, 2008). These might include spouses or significant others, parents, grandparents, brothers, sisters, and children.

When someone is injured or ill, that person's family members also suffer. This is especially true when the patient's condition is severe or life-threatening. The family members' stress, mental fatigue, and physical fatigue might be particularly acute in a hospital setting—especially when they first encounter their ill or injured loved one. But it remains serious after the fact, too, when they must care for their patient at home—especially if the condition is long-term or permanent. Indeed, research shows that 56% of caregivers reported feeling over-burdened and experiencing mental health problems (de Goumoëns, Marques Rio, & Ramelet, 2018). Not surprisingly, all this can make family members difficult for healthcare workers to deal with.

> ☑ **NOTE** Even the strongest families can become dysfunctional when a loved one faces a medical crisis (Boyd, 2008). Overwhelming stress combined with a lack of coping skills can trigger a dysfunctional state. Fortunately, these families usually return to normal functioning after the crisis passes.

At times, you will be called on to comfort and console family members who are overwhelmed with grief and stress. With every interaction, you can provide reassurance and emotional support (de Goumoëns et al., 2018). You might do this by offering a meal tray to a daughter sitting with her terminally ill parent or bringing up a cot for a fatigued father spending the night with an inpatient sick child. You can also encourage family members to talk to come to grips with their emotions, and to listen when they do (Wright & Leahey, 2013). This is itself a form of de-escalation.

> ☑ **NOTE** When dealing with a patient's family members, it is important to communicate support and compassion—especially when those family members are struggling to cope with a crisis.

In addition to providing emotional support, your core role in family care is to provide education. This includes education in behavioral management—including de-escalation—in a home setting. As part of holistic care, you should teach family members and caregivers how to prevent escalation and share de-escalation techniques. This provides them with a broader ability to manage behavioral issues that may arise in the home setting. It may also be beneficial to educate family members and caregivers on how to access your community's mental health system—for example, through the emergency department or through a community mental health clinic—if emergency mental health treatment is needed after discharge.

Online Resources for Families and Caregivers

▪ **Family Caregiver Alliance.** https://www.caregiver.org/

▪ **Alzheimer's Association: What Is Dementia?** https://www.alz.org/alzheimers-dementia/what-is-dementia

▪ **National Institute on Aging: Alzheimer's Disease and Related Dementias Portal.** https://www.nia.nih.gov/health/alzheimers

▪ **American Psychological Association Caregiving Resources.** https://www.apa.org/pi/about/publications/caregivers/resources/index

REFERENCES

American Psychiatric Association, American Psychiatric Nurses Association, & National Association of Psychiatric Health Systems. (2007). *Learning from each other: Success stories and ideas for reducing restraint/seclusion in behavioral health.* Retrieved from http://www.restraintfreeworld.org/documents/Learning%20From%20Each%20Other.pdf

Boyd, M. A. (2008). *Psychiatric nursing: Contemporary practice* (4th ed.). Philadelphia, PA: Lippincott, Williams & Wilkins.

Caplan, G. (1970). *The theory and practice of mental health consultation.* New York, NY: Basic Books, Inc.

Chou, K. R., Kaas, M. J., & Richie, M. F. (1996). Assaultive behavior in geriatric patients. *Journal of Gerontological Nursing, 22*(11), 31–38.

Cowin, L., Davies, R., Estall, G., Berlin, T., Fitzgerald, M., & Hoot, S. (2003). De-escalating aggression and violence in the mental health setting. *International Journal of Mental Health Nursing, 12*(1), 64–73.

de Goumoëns, V., Marques Rio, L., & Ramelet, A. S. (2018). Family-oriented interventions for adults with acquired brain injury and their families: A scoping review protocol. *JBI Database of Systemic Reviews and Implementation Reports, 16*(3), 635–641. doi: 10.11124/JBISRIR-2017-003410

The Joint Commission. (2019). *2019 comprehensive accreditation manual for hospitals.* Oak Brook, IL: Joint Commission.

Littrell, K. H., & Littrell, S. H. (1998). Current understanding of violence and aggression: Assessment and treatment. *Journal of Psychosocial Nursing and Mental Health Services, 36*(12), 18–24.

The National Institute for Occupational Safety and Health. (n.d.) *Occupational violence.* Retrieved from https://www.cdc.gov/niosh/topics/violence/default.html

Owen, C., Tarantello, C., Jones, M., & Tennant, C. (1998). Violence and aggression in psychiatric units. *Psychiatric Services, 49*(11), 1,452–1,457.

Patel, M. X., Sethi, F. N., Barnes, T. R., Dix, R., Dratcu, L., Fox, B., … Woods, L. (2018). Joint BAP NAPICU evidence-based consensus guidelines for the clinical management of acute disturbance: De-escalation and rapid tranquillisation. *Journal of Psychopharmacology, 32*(6), 601–640. doi: 10.1177/0269881118776738

Richmond, J. S., Berlin, J. S., Fishkind, A. B., Holloman, G. H., Zeller, S. L., Wilson, M. P., …
Ng, A. T. (2012). Verbal de-escalation of the agitated patient: Consensus statement of the American
Association for Emergency Psychiatry Project BETA De-Escalation Workgroup. *Western Journal of
Emergency Medicine, 13*(1), 17–25. doi: 10.5811/westjem.2011.9.6864

Snorrason, J., & Biering, P. (2018). The attributes of successful de-escalation and restraint teams.
International Journal of Mental Health Nursing, 27(6), 1842–1850. doi: 10.1111/inm.12493

Wright, L., & Leahey, M. (2013). *Nurses and families* (6th ed.). Philadelphia, PA: F.A. Davis Company.

2

VARIABLES AND RISK FACTORS FOR AGGRESSION

"Peace cannot be kept by force; it can only be achieved by understanding."

–Albert Einstein

OBJECTIVES

- Identify patient variables

- Describe environmental variables

- Examine caregiver variables

- Discuss patient and caregiver interaction variables

- Cover other key risk factors

Aggression is defined as harsh physical or verbal actions with the intent to harm another physically or mentally (Townsend, 2015). Unchecked aggression can escalate to violence. *Violence* is an outburst of physical force that abuses, injures, or harms another individual or object (Sunderland, 1997).

There is robust evidence to suggest that aggression and violence are associated with several variables and risk factors. The variables are as follows:

- Patient variables

- Environmental variables

- Caregiver risk factor (nursing and mental health staff) variables

- Patient and caregiver interaction variables

It is critical to recognize aggression early so you can implement de-escalation techniques immediately. In this way it is possible to break the escalation chain and prevent violence (Distasio, 1994; Littrell & Littrell, 1998; Sunderland, 1997; Swanson, 2008). Knowing these variables is critical to ensuring this early recognition and for helping prevent patients from engaging in aggressive behaviors in all forms toward self and others. So too is identifying other key risk factors related to aggression and violence.

The Origins of Violence

History tells us that human life in centuries past was often nasty, violent, brutish, and short—but that might not have always been so. Demeo (1991) offers substantial proof that our ancestors were peaceful, nonviolent, and far more social than they are today. Demeo contends that climate change around 4000 BCE brought hardship, famine, starvation, and migrations. This forced humans into violent social patterns due to competition for scarce resources for basic survival. In other words, violence is *not* natural to the human species (Pinker, 2011) and does *not* arise from the human character. It is an aberrant form of behavior for the human species. Studies of primates also show that both violent behavior and peaceful behavior are learned (Copeland-Linder, Lambert, & Ialongo, 2013; Sapolsky, 2007).

PATIENT VARIABLES

There are several patient variables associated with aggression. These include observable behaviors such as agitation, restlessness, anger, and lack of organization. Other patient variables include the following (Barlow, Grenyer, & Ilkiw-Lavalle, 2000; Chou, Kaas, & Richie, 1996; Hamrin, Iennaco, & Olsen, 2009):

▣ Mental instability

▣ The presence of delusions

▣ The presence of command hallucinations with violent content

▣ Poor impulse control

▣ Irritability

▣ Attention-seeking behavior

▣ An agitated state

▣ Disorganized thought processes

Some patient variables are considered particularly high-risk. These include the following:

▣ Carrying objects that could be used as weapons

▣ Progressive psychomotor agitation such as pacing

▣ Paranoid symptoms such as delusions of persecution

▣ Substance intoxication or withdrawal from alcohol or drugs (Johnson & Delaney, 2007; Rueve & Welton, 2008)

▣ Allergic reactions to medication or medication toxicity (Owen, Tarantello, Jones, & Tennant, 1998a)

Patients who carry the greatest risk for harmful intent are those who issue a planned or detailed threat of violence (Glasser, 1997; Hodgins, 2008). If the patient has an available means for inflicting injury, such as access to or ownership of a weapon, it is the most imminent indicator of risk of lethal intent to inflict harm on another (Franz, Zeh, Schablon, Kuhnert, & Nienhaus, 2010). On a related note, the best single predictor of aggression is a past history of violence—including animal cruelty. Individuals with a history of aggressive or violent behavior often inflict violence throughout their lives (Owen, Tarantello, Jones, & Tennant, 1998b). A recent act of violence is especially concerning. Other top indicators include a history of abuse and criminal behavior (Kleespies, 1998).

> ☑ **NOTE** The most common predictor of assaultive behavior is a history of assaultive behavior. Forty-three percent of assaultive patients are repeaters of violent acts. And, more than 77% of violent acts are perpetrated by individuals with a history of violence (Quanbeck et al., 2007).

When a person exhibits one of these indicators *and* poor impulse control, there's even more tendency to act out.

> ☑ **NOTE** Statistics indicate that young men with substance abuse issues are more likely to commit violence. So too are young men who are both uneducated and unemployed (Kleespies, 1998). Belonging to a demographic group with an increased prevalence of violence increases the violence risk (Chou et al., 1996; Hamrin et al., 2009).

ENVIRONMENTAL VARIABLES

For many patients, receiving healthcare services in general is experienced as stressful. So too is experiencing the discomfort of ill health and being inpatient in any hospital (Beattie, Griffith, Innes, & Morphet, 2019). Add to these environmental variables in healthcare venues, and the risk of aggressive behavior in some individuals increases substantially. Examples of environmental variables associated with aggressive behavior include the following:

- **Excessive motion.** Too much motion—for example, people constantly walking by—can agitate patients (Chou et al., 1996).

- **Excessive noxious noise.** Inpatient healthcare facilities are often noisy due to general everyday commotion. Environmental modifications such as internal renovations or construction can also produce noise. This noise can trigger aggression in individuals who are unable to cope with the constant clamor (Chou et al., 1996; Rueve & Welton, 2008).

- **Lack of stimulation.** Just as environments with excessive stimuli, like too much motion or noise, can cause aggression, so can environments that don't have enough stimuli, such as recreational and diversional activities (Cole, 2005; Johnson & Delaney, 2007).

- **Ever-changing inpatient populations.** Environments become unpredictable with the introduction of new patients. This can result in agitation.

- **The unpredictable behavior of others.** Staff or other patients who behave in unpredictable ways can trigger aggression.

- **Crowded inpatient facilities.** Crowded facilities may trigger aggressive behavior (Cole, 2005). For example, cramped accommodations or a noisy roommate could be cause for aggression. So too might a conflict between several patients over what television show to watch in the common area.

- **Locked unit.** Being an inpatient in a locked mental health unit, without the freedom to leave or to return home (e.g., due to involuntary admission), can trigger anger, aggression, and violence in some people—especially those with psychosis.

- **Chaos during meals and shift changes.** The most common times for inpatient violence are at meal times, when patients have eating utensils handy; and during shift changes, when the smallest number of staff are available on the unit.

- **Lack of privacy.** Many inpatients share rooms, bathrooms, and shower facilities, resulting in a feeling of a lack of privacy. Open-backed hospital gowns that have inadequate coverage of the patient's body can also result in this feeling. This can trigger aggression in some patients (Negley & Manley, 1990).

- **Lack of personal space.** The buffer zone of people who are prone to violence is four times larger than that of people who are not so inclined (Chou, Lu, & Mao, 2002; Giarelli et al., 2018; Negley & Manley, 1990). If that zone is violated, it could cause aggressive behavior.

> ✅ **NOTE** In more than 50% of cases of physical assault by patients in a healthcare facility, a caregiver violated the patient's personal space immediately before the attack.

- **A high influx of new admissions requiring acute complex medical care.** This is especially true with new male patients and with involuntary patients who are in treatment due to a court order.

- **Lack of dignity.** Suffering from an illness, and the accompanying hospitalization—during which time doctors and nurses often control the patient's healthcare decisions—can diminish one's sense of dignity. So can needing assistance with even simple everyday tasks such as walking to the bathroom or combing one's hair. This could cause some patients to feel disempowered and angry.

- **Lack of freedom or autonomy.** Patients who lack freedom and autonomy—including the ability to make decisions about their care—may become aggressive (Johnson & Delaney, 2007; Lehmann, McCormick, & Kizer, 1999).

- **Lack of structure.** If there's no predictable schedule in the healthcare environment, there is an increased risk of aggressive behavior (Johnson & Delaney, 2007).

The bottom line: A poor environment that contains significant stressors is one of the most common causes of aggression and violence on inpatient mental health units. Fortunately, it's possible to address these issues. It is critical to provide a safe environment for everyone.

CAREGIVER VARIABLES

There are many caregiver variables that influence the frequency of inpatient aggression. Here are several examples:

- **Staff educational level.** Research has revealed a correlation between inpatient aggression and healthcare staff education (Barlow et al., 2000). The higher the educational nursing level, the lower the risk of encountering violence. Nurse aides and nursing students are at the highest risk of physical assault.

- **Lack of training in de-escalation and aggression management.** This prevents healthcare staff from recognizing escalating behaviors, engaging in early intervention, and using effective de-escalation skills to defuse the aggression (Chou et al., 2002; Cowin et al., 2003).

- **Staff skills and work experience.** The healthcare staff members most likely to encounter aggression are new nurses and nurses lacking experience in de-escalation techniques (Lanza, Kayne, Hicks, & Milner, 1991). In contrast, experienced nurses have likely developed skills to prevent aggression and defuse agitated patients, resulting in fewer assaultive encounters.

- **Lack of familiarity with the venue of care.** Sometimes nurses and other healthcare staff are new employees or have been pulled to the unit from another area of the hospital and are unfamiliar with the unit's environment and patients. This can cause major stress for staff and patients, which can trigger both anger and aggression.

- **Lack of familiarity with the patient.** When healthcare staff are caring for a patient for the first time—either because the staff are new to the unit or the patient is—they might not be familiar with that patient's particular care needs or how best to de-escalate the patient if aggression results.

- **Rigidity of routines.** When nursing staff place greater emphasis on maintaining institutional routines, there is often a rise in violence (Distasio, 1994; Simon & Tardiff, 2008). In inflexible environments, staff often overreact to uncooperative patients, which can provoke assault.

- **Excessive physical limits.** Assaults frequently occur while staff members are placing a patient in a restraint or administering medication. Healthcare staff should avoid this practice unless there is a clear need to protect the patient or others. Instead of setting physical limits, it's better to set behavioral limits. This can be as easy as telling the patient, "No hitting or hurting is allowed here," or "You are a partner in keeping this environment safe for yourself and for other people." When setting behavioral limits, use specific and direct language. Tell the patient what you expect and the consequences if those expectations are not met. (For best results, speak with the patient one-on-one in a quiet area.)

- **Lack of therapeutic communication skills among nurses.** Nurses who lack therapeutic communication skills have a reduced ability to verbally de-escalate agitated patients before they lose self-control.

- **An aloof or uncaring manner.** Nurses with a poor demeanor communicate a lack of caring and a lack of respect. This may trigger agitation or aggression in some patients (Lion, Synder, & Merrill, 1981).

- **A lack of emotional and physical availability.** When patients notice that the only time a nurse talks to them is when they act out, they learn that they must act out to get the nurse's attention. To prevent this, nurses must make themselves available to patients. Research shows that when nurses offer availability, they encounter less aggression on the unit (Hamrin et al., 2009; Lanza et al., 1991). Offering availability also conveys caring and empathy. This helps develop therapeutic rapport, which in turn prevents aggression and potential violence.

> ☑ **NOTE** Patients need to know they can to talk to a nurse in a nonthreat-
> ening environment. Making the patient aware that nurses are always avail-
> able to listen imparts caring, establishes therapeutic rapport, and prevents
> violence.

PATIENT AND CAREGIVER INTERACTION VARIABLES

Variables can also arise from interactions between patients and caregivers.
Research indicates that more than 56% of inpatient assaults resulted from
patient-staff conflict (Chou et al., 2002). The most common of these conflicts are
power struggles. Nurses should avoid power struggles whenever possible because
they are a frequent catalyst for violence. Instead of engaging in power struggles
with patients, partner with them to provide collaborative, holistic, patient-
centered care.

Other interaction variables include nurses who have "high expressed emotion"
(such as a loud, high-pitched, or shrill tone of voice), who show high levels of
anxiety, or who are prone to overreaction. Always speak to patients in a pleasant,
calm, professional voice. Finally, placing too many demands on a patient may
cause feelings of powerlessness and trigger agitation (Hamrin et al., 2009; Lanza
et al., 1991).

> ☑ **NOTE** In mental health nursing, we know that operating one day at a
> time—even one moment at a time—is the best way to deliver safe, holistic
> care. Allow patients to make choices and decisions about their care. Give
> patients time and space to meet their needs and to establish a trusting
> therapeutic rapport with their caregiver.

OTHER RISK FACTORS

In addition to the variables discussed, there are other risk factors for aggression. For example, threats to self-concept, overwhelming stress, suspicion of
others, paranoid ideation, delusions, command hallucinations, hostility, and rage
increase the risk of aggressiveness toward others (Moyer, 1968). Another risk
factor is brain injury.

This section focuses on risk factors that relate to certain mental disorders. (A few of these were mentioned in the "Patient Variables" section earlier in this chapter.) These include (in order of frequency) psychotic disorders, organic disorders, and personality disorders. Of course, the severity of these disorders affects how likely it is that an individual suffering from one of them will become aggressive (Distasio, 1994). (Specific de-escalation interventions for members of these high-risk groups are discussed later in this book.)

> ☑ **NOTE** Early intervention is especially important when dealing with individuals in these high-risk groups. The earlier the intervention, the greater the chances it will be effective in restoring a calm state.

The following psychotic disorders may result in aggressive behavior (Hodgins, 2008; Simon & Tardiff, 2008):

- **Schizophrenia.** People who suffer from schizophrenia sometimes experience altered perceptions of reality such as hallucinations and delusions (American Psychiatric Association [APA], 2013; Hamrin et al., 2009). This could cause them to engage in aggressive behavior toward others. This is particularly true for people with paranoid schizophrenia. These individuals may sometimes hear "voices"—the most frequent form of auditory hallucination (Kane, 2003). Frequently, these voices command patients to harm themselves or others. People suffering from schizophrenia are also at a high risk for self-harming aggressive behaviors up to and including suicide.

> ❗ **CAUTION** Patients suffering from command hallucinations are four times more likely to harm themselves or others—meaning you may need to take precautions to protect them and those around them from harm. Always complete an in-depth assessment of any auditory hallucinations a patient reports.

- **Bipolar disorder.** Like people with schizophrenia, individuals with bipolar disorder my experience altered perceptions of reality and engage in self-harming behaviors, with the same negative outcomes. The mania associated with bipolar disorder may also trigger aggressive behavior; so too can the dysfunctional grief experienced by bipolar patients (Chou et al., 2002; Khalsa, Baldessarini, Tohen, & Salvatore, 2018).

> ☑ **NOTE** Schizophrenia and bipolar disorder account for a large percentage of inpatient assaults. The majority of inpatient violence is associated with a primary diagnosis of schizophrenia (62%) and bipolar disorder (24.6%) (Chou et al., 2002; Falk et al., 2014). These patients become assaultive due to impulsiveness, delusions, hallucinations, and disorganized thought processes.

Organic disorders are likewise associated with aggression and rapid escalation (Bowers et al., 2009; Hamrin et al., 2009)—though for different reasons. Organic disorders include:

- Brain injury
- Dementia
- Degenerative brain diseases such as Alzheimer's disease
- Organic brain syndrome (OBS)
- Delirium
- Substance abuse disorder
- Infections

Dementia, organic disorders with neuro-physiological deficit manifestations, and degenerative diseases like Alzheimer's may in and of themselves cause heightened aggressive behavior toward others due to a deterioration in mental function. For example, individuals with dementia often experience impaired cognition or confusion, which can cause them to become agitated (Chou et al., 1996). Some dementia patients also experience a phenomenon called sundowning, which describes a state of confusion that occurs late in the day and causes them to become aggressive.

With substance abuse disorder, it is often disinhibition and loss of control that increase the risk of agitation and violent behavior (APA, 2013). People suffering from substance abuse disorder might also exhibit aggression during withdrawal, especially from stimulants such as cocaine, methamphetamines, and club drugs such as bath salts (Varghese, Khakha, & Chadda, 2016). Finally, people suffering from substance abuse disorder often exhibit aggressively manipulative behavior, are accusatory, and have antisocial characteristics.

As for infections, these often result in confusion, particularly among the elderly. As with patients suffering from dementia, this feeling of confusion can lead to agitated behavior—especially in response to misinterpreted environmental stimuli.

Borderline personality disorder is one personality disorder that is associated with increased risk of agitated or violent behavior (Hamrin et al., 2009; New, Tucci, & Rios, 2017; Umhau, Trandem, Shah, & George, 2012; Vieta et al., 2017). Symptoms of borderline personality disorder include poor impulse control and an inability to control one's emotions. Patients who suffer from this condition may therefore become easily agitated and can quickly escalate to aggressive and even out-of-control behavior toward others. So might patients who suffer from other personality disorders such as impulse control disorder and paranoid personality disorder.

Other mental disorders associated with aggression are antisocial personality disorder, conduct disorder, delusional disorder, depression, and intermittent explosive disorder. In addition, anxiety disorders can quickly escalate to acute panic levels. When this happens, as the patient's fear increases, so too does the likelihood of aggressive behavior.

> ✅ **NOTE** Psychosis, anxiety, and depression are leading causes of aggression, especially among the elderly (Desai & Grossberg, 2001; Hall, Hall, & Chapman, 2009).

> ✅ **NOTE** The risk of aggression and violence increases if patients do not adhere to their prescribed psychiatric medication regimen or abruptly stop taking the medication on their own (Gillespie, Gates, Miller, & Howard, 2010). With some psychiatric medications, it's imperative that patients taper down their use over time and under the care of a trained physician or psychiatrist rather than quitting them "cold turkey." Otherwise the patient could experience withdrawal symptoms that result in aberrant, agitated, or aggressive behavior (Boyd, 2008).

Finally, hereditary factors can increase the risk of aggression, as can biochemical alterations in the brain. Genetic research studies are underway to determine whether there are genetic markers or a specific genetic mutation that drives anger and aggressive behavior. This could lead to breakthroughs in the treatment of disorders associated with aggression (Kneisl & Trigoboff, 2009; Meyer et al., 2018).

Figure 2.1 shows several common conditions that could indicate a higher risk of aggression. Figure 2.2 shows how the variables and other risk factors combine to spark aggressive behavior in some patients.

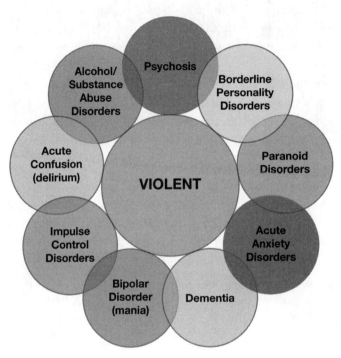

FIGURE 2.1 Conditions commonly associated with an increased risk of aggression.

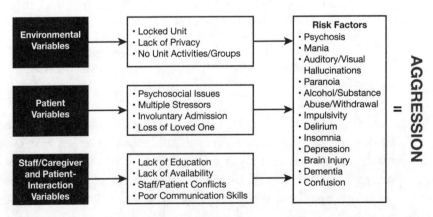

FIGURE 2.2 Combining variables and risk factors can have explosive results.

REFERENCES

American Psychiatric Association. (2013). *Diagnostic and statistical manual of mental disorders (DSM-5)*. Washington, DC: American Psychiatric Association.

Barlow, K., Grenyer, B., & Ilkiw-Lavalle, O. (2000). Prevalence and precipitants of aggression in psychiatric inpatient units. *Australian and New Zealand Journal of Psychiatry, 34*(6), 967–974.

Beattie, J., Griffith, D., Innes, K., & Morphet, J. (2019). Workplace violence perpetrated by clients of health care: A need for safety and trauma-informed care. *Journal of Clinical Nursing, 28*(1–2), 116–124. doi: 10.1111/jocn.14683

Bowers, L., Allan, T., Simpson, A., Jones, J., van der Merwe, M., & Jeffery, D. (2009). Identifying key factors associated with aggression in acute inpatient psychiatric wards. *Issues in Mental Health Nursing, 30*(4), 260–271. doi: 10.1080/01612840802710829

Boyd, M. A. (2008). *Psychiatric nursing: Contemporary practice* (4th ed.). Philadelphia, PA: Lippincott, Williams & Wilkins.

Chou, K. R., Kaas, M. J., & Richie, M. F. (1996). Assaultive behavior in geriatric patients. *Journal of Gerontological Nursing, 22*(11), 31–38.

Chou, K. R., Lu, R. B., & Mao, W. C. (2002). Factors relevant to patient assaultive behavior and assault in acute inpatient psychiatric units in Taiwan. *Archives of Psychiatric Nursing, 16*(4), 187–195.

Cole, A. (2005). Four in five nurses on mental wards face violence. *British Medical Journal, 330*(7502), 1227.

Copeland-Linder, N., Lambert, S. F., & Ialongo, N. S. (2013). Community violence, protective factors, and adolescent mental health: A profile analysis. *Journal of Child & Adolescent Psychology, 39*(2), 176–186. doi: 10.1080/15374410903532601

Cowin, L., Davies, R., Estall, G., Berlin, T., Fitzgerald, M., & Hoot, S. (2003). De-escalating aggression and violence in the mental health setting. *International Journal of Mental Health Nursing, 12*(1), 64–73.

Demeo, J. (1991). The origins and diffusion of patrism in Saharasia, c.4000 BCE: Evidence for a worldwide, climate-linked geographical pattern in human behavior. *World Futures, 30*(4), 247–271.

Desai, A. K., & Grossberg, G. T. (2001). Recognition and management of behavioral disturbances in dementia. *The Primary Care Companion to the Journal of Clinical Psychiatry, 3*(3), 93–109.

Distasio, C. A. (1994). Violence in health care: Institutional strategies to cope with the phenomenon. *Health Care Supervisor, 12*(4), 1–34.

Falk, O., Wallinius, M., Lundström, S., Frisell, T., Anckarsäter, H., & Kerekes, N. (2014). The 1% of the population accountable for 63% of all violent crime convictions. *Social Psychiatry and Psychiatric Epidemiology, 49*(4), 559–571. doi: 10.1007/s00127-013-0783-y

Franz, S., Zeh, A., Schablon, A., Kuhnert, S., & Nienhaus, A. (2010). Aggression and violence against health care workers in Germany—A cross sectional retrospective survey. *BMC Health Services Research, 10*, 51. doi: 10.1186/1472-6963-10-51

Giarelli, E., Nocera, R., Jobes, M., Boylan, C., Lopez, J., & Knerr, J. (2018). Exploration of aggression/violence among adult patients admitted for short-term, acute-care mental health services. *Archives of Psychiatric Nursing, 32*(2), 215–223. doi: 10.1016/j.apnu.2017.11.004

Gillespie, G. L., Gates, D. M., Miller, M., & Howard, P. K. (2010). Workplace violence in healthcare settings: Risk factors and protective strategies. *Rehabilitation Nursing, 35*(5), 177–184.

Glasser, W. (1997). *Violence and aggression: Assessing risk, affecting outcomes.* Philadelphia, PA: Brunner/Mazel.

Hall, Ryan C. W., Hall, Richard C. W., & Chapman, M. J. (2009). Nursing home violence: Occurrence, risks, and interventions. *Annals of Long-Term Care, 17*(1).

Hamrin, V., Iennaco, J., & Olsen, D. (2009). A review of ecological factors affecting inpatient psychiatric unit violence: Implications for relational and unit cultural improvements. *Issues in Mental Health Nursing, 30*(4), 214–226. doi: 10.1080/01612840802701083

Hodgins, S. (2008). Violent behaviour among people with schizophrenia: A framework for investigations of causes, and effective treatment, and prevention. *Philosophical Transactions of the Royal Society of London, Series B, Biological Sciences, 363*(1503), 2,505–2,518. doi: 10.1098/rstb.2008.0034

Johnson, M. E., & Delaney, K. R. (2007). Keeping the unit safe: The anatomy of escalation. *Journal of the American Psychiatric Nurses Association, 13*(1), 42–50.

Kane, J. M. (2003). Review of treatments that can ameliorate nonadherence in patients with schizophrenia. *The Journal of Clinical Psychology, 67*(Suppl. 5), 9–14.

Khalsa, H. K., Baldessarini, R. J., Tohen, M., & Salvatore, P. (2018). Aggression among 216 patients with a first-psychotic episode of bipolar I disorder. *International Journal of Bipolar Disorders, 6*(1), 18.

Kleespies, P. M. (1998). *Emergencies in mental health practice.* New York, NY: Guilford Press.

Kneisl, C. R., & Trigoboff, E. (2009). *Contemporary psychiatric-mental health nursing* (2nd ed.). Upper Saddle River, NJ: Prentice Hall.

Lanza, M. L., Kayne, H. L., Hicks, C., & Milner, J. (1991). Nursing staff characteristics related to patient assault. *Issues in Mental Health Nursing, 12*(3), 253–265.

Lehmann, L. S., McCormick, R. A., & Kizer, K. W. (1999). A survey of assaultive behavior in Veterans Health Administrative facilities. *Psychiatric Services, 50*(3), 384–389.

Lion, J. R., Synder, W., & Merrill, G. L. (1981). Underreporting of assaults on staff in a state hospital. *Hospital and Community Psychiatry, 32*(7), 497–498.

Littrell, K. H., & Littrell, S. H. (1998). Current understanding of violence and aggression: Assessment and treatment. *Journal of Psychosocial Nursing and Mental Health Services, 36*(12), 18–24.

Meyer, L. F., Telles, L. E. B., Mecler, K., Soares, A. L. A. G., Alves, R. S., & Valença, A. M. (2018). Schizophrenia and violence: Study in a general psychiatric hospital with HCR-20 and MOAS. *Trends in Psychiatry and Psychotherapy, 40*(4), 310–317. doi: 10.1590/2237-6089-2017-0039

Moyer, K. E. (1968). Kinds of aggression and their physiological basis. *Communications in Behavioral Biology, 2*(2), 65–87.

Negley, E. N., & Manley, J. T. (1990). Environmental interventions in assaultive behavior. *Journal of Gerontological Nursing, 16*(3), 29–33.

New, A., Tucci, V. T., & Rios, J. (2017). A modern-day fight club? The stabilization and management of acutely agitated patients in the emergency department. *The Psychiatric Clinics of North America, 40*(3), 397–410. doi: 10.1016/j.psc.2017.05.002

Owen, C., Tarantello, C., Jones, M., & Tennant, C. (1998a). Repetitively violent patients in psychiatric units. *Psychiatric Services, 49*(11), 1458–1461.

Owen, C., Tarantello, C., Jones, M., & Tennant, C. (1998b). Violence and aggression in psychiatric units. *Psychiatric Services, 49*(11), 1452–1457.

Pinker, S. (2011). *The better angels of our nature: Why violence has declined.* New York, NY: Viking Books.

Quanbeck, C. D., McDermott, B. E., Lam, J., Eisenstark, H., Sokolov, G., & Scott, C. L. (2007). Categorization of aggressive acts committed by chronically assaultive state hospital patients. *Psychiatric Services, 58*(4), 521–528.

Rueve, M. E., & Welton, R. S. (2008). Violence and mental illness. *Psychiatry, 5*(5), 34–48.

Sapolsky, R. M. (2007, September 1). Peace among primates. *Greater Good Magazine.* Retrieved from https://greatergood.berkeley.edu/article/item/peace_among_primates

Simon, R. I., & Tardiff, K. (2008). *Textbook of violence assessment and management.* St. Louis, MO: American Psychiatric Publishing, Inc.

Sunderland, T. (1997). The diagnosis and epidemiology of violence and agitation. *American Psychiatric Association, 278*(16), 1,363–1,371.

Swanson, J. W. (2008). Preventing the unpredicted: Managing violence risk in mental health care. *Psychiatric Services, 59*(2), 191–193. doi: 10.1176/ps.2008.59.2.191

Townsend, M. C. (2015). *Psychiatric mental health nursing: Concepts of care in evidence-based practice* (8th ed.). Philadelphia, PA: F. A. Davis Company.

Umhau, J. C., Trandem, K., Shah, M., & George, D. T. (2012). The physician's unique role in preventing violence: A neglected opportunity? *BMC Medicine, 10,* 146.

Varghese, A., Khakha, D. C., & Chadda, R. K. (2016). Pattern and type of aggressive behavior in patients with severe mental illness as perceived by the caregivers and the coping strategies used by them in a tertiary care hospital. *Archives of Psychiatric Nursing, 30*(1), 62–69. doi: 10.1016/j.apnu.2015.10.002

Vieta, E., Garriga, M., Cardete, L., Bernardo, M., Lombraña, M., Blanch, J., … Martínez-Arán, A. (2017). Protocol for the management of psychiatric patients with psychomotor agitation. *BioMedCentral Psychiatry, 17*(1), 328. doi: 10.1186/s12888-017-1490-0

3

ASSESSING AN ESCALATING SITUATION FOR EARLY INTERVENTION

"Darkness cannot drive out darkness: Only light can do that. Hate cannot drive out hate; only love can do that."

–Dr. Martin Luther King, Jr.

OBJECTIVES

- Explore the aggression continuum and escalation cycle
- Map out the assault cycle
- Identify triggers of aggressive or violent behavior
- Identify escalating behaviors
- Assess the patient's behavior for signs of agitation
- Grasp the importance of early intervention

In any tense situation, assessment is a critical practice. Correctly assessing a situation enables you to determine whether escalation has occurred or is likely to occur and to quickly intervene. Based on your assessment, you can develop strategies to de-escalate the situation. That's what this chapter is about. It discusses the aggression continuum and the escalation cycle, identifies common causes of escalation and common escalation behaviors, and discusses the importance of early intervention.

THE AGGRESSION CONTINUUM AND THE ESCALATION CYCLE

Tense situations often escalate into incidents involving aggression. *Aggression* is defined as an intense physical or verbal reaction that indicates rage. Aggression may in turn escalate to physical or verbal destruction that can harm self or others (Simon & Tardiff, 2008).

The escalation of aggression occurs on a continuum. Absent the initiation of de-escalation interventions, the aggression will likely progress along the continuum. As it does, anxiety and emotion are heightened, and anger is often the result. Being aware of this continuum can help you correctly assess a tense situation.

As shown in Figure 3.1, this continuum has three phases:

1. **The trigger phase.** In this phase, a catalyst event that causes stress starts the escalation process (Byrnes, 2000).

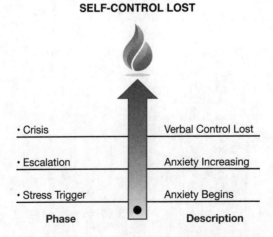

FIGURE 3.1 Loss of self-control into violence.

2. **The escalation phase.** During this stage, anxiety builds, arousing angry emotions.

3. **The crisis phase.** In this phase, the person loses control of the ability to speak and eventually experiences a total loss of reason and self-control (Byrnes, 2000). An individual may act violently toward others in this phase.

As individuals progress through the aggression continuum, their emotions often escalate in a predictable cycle (see Figure 3.2):

1. **Calm.** Individuals are in this stage before a catalyst event triggers them.

2. **Anxious.** This stage occurs after a triggering event. People in this stage of the cycle may exhibit behaviors such as a tense posture, fidgeting, pacing, hand-wringing, foot-tapping, and irritability. They rarely verbalize their anxiety, choosing to bottle it up instead. This sometimes causes them to explode—quickly advancing from anxiety through the remaining phases of the cycle.

3. **Agitated.** As the situation escalates, the person may become agitated. Behavioral signs of agitation may include clenching one's teeth or fists, cursing, and shouting.

4. **Aggressive.** An aggressive person might display any number of telling behaviors. These might include insulting, intimidating, or threatening other patients or staff; slamming doors; violating the rights, personal space, or privacy of others; and destroying property—for example, breaking chairs, ripping out wires, or destroying wall hangings or other objects (Cowin et al., 2003).

5. **Violent.** There are many manifestations of violent behavior. These include harming behaviors such as striking, punching, slapping, biting, and hair-pulling. Throwing objects at others in an attempt to injure them is also considered violent behavior.

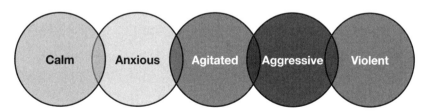

FIGURE 3.2 The cycle of escalation.

Early intervention is key. It's far better—and far easier—to de-escalate a situation involving someone who is anxious than one involving someone who is violent. It is imperative to begin de-escalation efforts at the first signs of anxiety. This breaks the chain of escalation.

> ☑ **NOTE** There is a broad window of opportunity between these stages to recognize escalation and to intervene using de-escalation techniques to defuse agitation and prevent physical violence.

Of course, it may not always be possible to intervene early. In that case it's important to know that different stages in the cycle of escalation require different de-escalation techniques. Table 3.1 reviews the four stages of the cycle that require intervention and associated behaviors and suggests de-escalation techniques you can use—a sort of "de-escalation algorithm." (Chapter 4, "De-Escalation Techniques," discusses some of these techniques in more detail.)

Safety First

In all four stages of the escalation cycle that require intervention, staff should put safety first—their own safety and that of the patient and others present. One way to do this is to open up lines of therapeutic communication with the agitated individual. Another is to avoid overreacting and to use the least restrictive intervention possible given the patient's behavior (Simon & Tardiff, 2008). If the situation escalates to the point where the patient becomes violent, it may be necessary to notify security or police. Behavioral emergency response teams are also available in many mental health and medical healthcare facilities to assist with de-escalation. For more on ensuring the safety of patients and those around them, see Chapter 17, "Staying Safe During De-Escalation."

TABLE 3.1 **The De-Escalation Algorithm**

Phase in Escalation Cycle	Associated Behaviors	Suggested De-Escalation Interventions
Anxious	Tense posture	Encourage verbalization.
	Fidgeting	Ask open-ended questions.
	Pacing	Offer a book or magazine.
	Hand-wringing	Move the patient to a quiet environment.
	Foot-tapping	Offer the patient a snack, a meal, or a beverage.
	Irritability	Encourage the patient to perform relaxation exercises.
	Nail-biting	Put on some pleasant music.
		Decrease stressors.
Agitated	Clenched teeth	Encourage verbalization.
	Clenched fists	Ask open-ended questions.
	Cursing	Offer to help.
	Shouting	Find and resolve the issue.
	Red face	Assess for pain and administer pain medication if needed.
	Abrupt movements	Offer to help.
		Offer the patient a puzzle or game.
		Have the patient write in a journal.
		Have the patient perform progressive muscular relaxation exercises.
Aggressive	Issuing insults or threats	Redirect the patient.
	Intimidating others	Set limits.
	Slamming doors	Engage in therapeutic communication.
	Invading the rights, space, or privacy of others	Encourage verbalization.
		Ask open-ended questions.
	Destroying property	Offer choices.
	Grabbing	
Violent	Striking	Say "STOP."
	Punching	Open lines of communication.
	Slapping	Encourage cooperation.
	Biting	Administer PRN (as needed) medication.
	Hair-pulling	Call for assistance from staff, security, or police (depending on facility policy).
	Throwing objects at others	
	Kicking	

THE ASSAULT CYCLE

Caplan (1970) described an assault cycle with six key phases. Identifying which phase a patient is in is an important part of the assessment process. The phases are as follows:

1. **Activation.** In this first phase, the patient may exhibit body language that indicates agitation, such as pacing. Or, the patient might shout loudly at family members.

2. **Escalation.** During this phase, the patient begins to display more disruptive behavior, such as shouting, cursing, or making hostile or unreasonable demands.

3. **Crisis.** It is in this phase that the patient acts out in aggressive or violent ways—for example, shouting, striking out, or biting others.

4. **Recovery.** In this phase, de-escalation interventions have begun to take hold. The patient begins to get a grip on emotions and to regain self-control.

5. **Post-crisis depression.** After regaining control, the patient may feel embarrassed or remorseful about the incident and could become depressed or even despondent as a result. Patients in this phase may become teary and often apologize to staff for their actions.

6. **Stabilization.** In this phase, the patient has completely regained self-control. The patient has reestablished normal behavior and restored normal routine.

Of these phases, the first three—activation, escalation, and crisis—require specific de-escalation interventions by a healthcare professional, if possible. Table 3.2 outlines what interventions you should use to manage each of these three phases. (For more on these interventions, see Chapter 4.)

TABLE 3.2 Managing the First Three Phases of the Assault Cycle

Phase	Common Patient Behaviors	Suggested Interventions
Activation	Pacing	Encourage verbalization.
	Shouting at family members	Offer to help.
	Finger-tapping	Provide comfort measures such as a warm blanket.
	Irritability	Offer a snack or beverage.
	Anxiousness	Re-orient the patient.
	Shrill voice	Move the patient to a quiet environment.

Phase	Common Patient Behaviors	Suggested Interventions
Escalation	Shouting	Encourage verbalization.
	Cursing	Redirect the patient.
	Making hostile or unreasonable demands	Eliminate stressors.
		Offer to help.
	Threats	Assist the patient in problem-solving.
	Clenched fists	Encourage the patient to perform relaxation exercises such as deep breathing.
	Clenched teeth	
	Violating personal space	
Crisis	Shouting	Encourage verbalization.
	Striking out	Establish rapport (or enlist help from another staff member who already has).
	Biting others	
	Slapping	Redirect the patient.
	Grabbing hair	Move the patient to a quiet environment (reduce noise).
	Kicking	
		Administer PRN medication as per physician/psychiatrist order.

Chabora, Judge-Gorny, & Grogan, 2003; Hilgers, 2003; Paterson, Leadbetter, & McComish, 1997

As mentioned, the last three phases are recovery, post-crisis depression, and stabilization. These require interventions that focus on helping patients regain emotional control and on debriefing to determine what happened and how the situation can be prevented in the future.

In the recovery phase, patients' tone of voice will become lower, and muscle tension will decrease. Their hands will unclench. They will begin to cooperate and follow instructions.

> **? TIP** During the recovery phase, it is beneficial for patients to have a quiet space in which to focus and to get a grip on their emotions. This will give them an opportunity to rationalize the situation and think through what has just happened. Deep breathing exercises will help the patients restore self-control and calm. Progressive muscular relaxation exercise is useful to relieve muscle tension and dissipate anger.

In the post-crisis depression phase, you might see patients holding their head in their hands. Or, they might be too embarrassed to make eye contact. They might cry. They might also apologize repeatedly. It is important in this phase to encourage the patients to verbalize their feelings. Listen to them in a caring, respectful manner and give emotional support.

In the stabilization phase, patients have been restored to their baseline normal behavior. They are calm and centered and have regained self-control. At this point, you should initiate a debriefing with the patients. In the first interaction of this debriefing, you should ask them if they are OK. Then gently encourage them to relate their view of what happened—including what caused the crisis. You should also ask the patients how the situation could have been handled differently to prevent it from happening again. The information from the patient debriefing is included in the treatment plan to prevent future aggressive episodes and for facility quality improvement.

TRIGGERS OF AGGRESSIVE OR VIOLENT BEHAVIOR

Any number of events, perceptions, or conditions can serve as triggers of aggressive or violent behavior. Obvious triggers include attempts to protect vital interests such as self-esteem and self-respect as well as drug or alcohol abuse. But these are far from the only triggers. Here are a few more to watch out for:

- **Sudden illness or hospitalization.** Suddenly finding oneself seriously injured or ill can trigger aggressive behavior in some patients.

- **Staff expectations.** If the staff on the unit treat the patients as if they will act out, then chances are they will do just that. To avoid this, begin each shift with a positive outlook. If you believe your patients will stay in control, then they probably will.

- **Staff behavior.** Some patients could become aggressive in response to a hostile or disrespectful staff member. To prevent this, healthcare providers must *always* be calm, caring, courteous, and kind. It is crucial to exhibit professional behavior and treat others as you would like to be treated.

> ☑ **NOTE** Respect is vital. Research indicates that a lack of respect is *the* main cause of most violence (Tingleff, Bradley, Gildberg, Munksgaard, & Hounsgaard, 2017). For best results in any intervention, you must show respect for the patient while also working to maintain the patient's dignity and autonomy (Lown & Setnik, 2018).

- **Lack of alternative methods of expression.** Some people only know how to express anger as physical aggression toward others. Research has shown, however, that when a person is taught how to verbalize anger, the risk of that person becoming aggressive is greatly reduced (Distasio, 1994). One way to encourage someone to verbalize anger is to simply ask open-ended questions, such as "What is upsetting you?"

- **Lack of personal space.** Violent people need more personal space than nonviolent people. In fact, people with a history of violence have been shown to require three to four times more personal space than non-aggressive people (Distasio, 1994). When communicating with an agitated person, therefore, you should step back and allow plenty of space. This will help to decrease the person's anxiety.

- **Loss of meaningful activity or sense of purpose.** Medical illness and long hospitalizations with nothing to do often result in endless boredom. This compounds the emotional trauma associated with an altered or diminished lifestyle. Nurses and other healthcare workers can counteract this by providing patients with plenty of diverse activities or by asking family members to bring in games or hobby supplies. This encourages meaningful engagement in the recovery process and provides educational opportunities for personal enlightenment and enhancement.

- **Increased frustration or confusion.** The disorientation and confusion that often accompanies medical illness can trigger frustration, fear, and anger—especially if patients are told they will be required to remain in the facility longer than expected. This is only made worse if patients are unable to recognize those around them or their surroundings (Hamrin, Iennaco, & Olsen, 2009).

- **Impaired communication.** Being unable to clearly voice their needs due to illness or injury can leave patients with overwhelming feelings of frustration and anger. To ameliorate this, provide writing materials for patients with voice impairment to aid in communication. On a related note, provide interpreters for deaf patients (Hamrin et al., 2009).

- **Diminished self-esteem.** Physical and mental limitations that result from chronic illness can damage self-esteem and self-confidence. To build self-esteem, address patients using their proper names; use Mr., Mrs.,

Miss, or Ms., or sir or ma'am. This shows respect. Also, never talk over the patient's head. Finally, when the patient speaks, listen respectfully, and offer a head nod or give verbal confirmation to convey your understanding.

- **Physical disability.** Physical disabilities, such as from a stroke or traumatic brain injury, may complicate recovery, causing the patient to become frustrated. For example, after a brain injury, some patients may need to relearn even the most basic skills, such as bathing and dressing themselves. Providing caring and compassionate care to these patients can prevent escalation. Also, when caring for those with a physical disability, make it a point to emphasize their abilities rather than their disabilities. For example, the first time they try to button their own shirt after suffering a traumatic brain injury, compliment them on the four buttons they got right instead of pointing out the one they missed. Provide positive reinforcement for what the patients can do, and you will promote more positive behaviors.

- **Physical pain.** Some people have trouble communicating when they are experiencing physical pain. This may cause them to become quite agitated. If you notice patients aggressively pacing around the unit, or if you know they have recently undergone surgery, ask if they are in pain. If the answer is yes, you may be able to de-escalate the situation quite easily by administering pain medication (Caplan, 1964).

Beware of Misunderstandings

Nurses like to converse at the nurses' station. Unfortunately, patients often overhear these conversations and assume they are about them—even when they aren't. This can cause patients to become agitated and angry.

If you are discussing anything that might be misinterpreted or is simply a volatile topic, it's best to move to the break room or any other area outside of hearing range for patients. Remember: In healthcare facilities, the walls have ears. Words can carry and be misunderstood. Nurses don't want to be placed in a de-escalation situation because patients were offended by remarks that were not even about them!

ESCALATING BEHAVIORS

Rarely will patients simply walk up to you and state that they feel agitated. You must be able to identify escalating behaviors on your own.

One way to identify escalating behaviors is through a person's body language. Here are several examples of body language behaviors that convey agitation. Being able to identify these early signs of agitation will enable you to intervene as quickly as possible, as well as observe when patients are beginning to calm down:

- An angry facial expression such as a frown or scowl
- Hand-wringing
- Standing in a corner or closed area
- Changes in breathing such as snorting or huffing and puffing
- A red face
- Distended neck veins
- A furrowed brow
- Clenching and unclenching of hands or teeth

In addition to body language, agitated patients might display more obvious or verbal signs of agitation or aggression. These could include the following:

- Mumbling to oneself
- Cursing or using other forceful words
- Using a harsh voice
- Shouting
- Large motor activity such as pacing, pounding one's palm with one's fist, or swinging one's arms about one's body (Caplan, 1964)
- Making demands or ordering others around
- Destroying property (even just throwing a pencil)
- Refusing to follow directions
- Intimidating others
- Boasting of past acts of violence
- Issuing verbal threats to peers or staff

Often these behaviors will occur in a progression, as shown in Figure 3.3. Too often, the end result is overt violence, such as biting or punching.

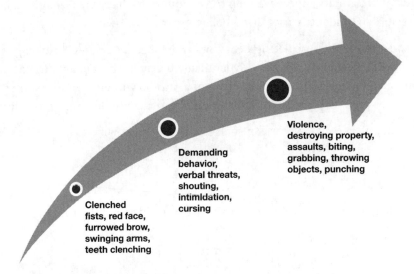

Violence, destroying property, assaults, biting, grabbing, throwing objects, punching

Demanding behavior, verbal threats, shouting, intimidation, cursing

Clenched fists, red face, furrowed brow, swinging arms, teeth clenching

FIGURE 3.3 A common progression of escalating behaviors.

If you notice any of these early behaviors, you must intervene immediately to prevent escalation and reduce the potential for violence (American Psychiatric Association, American Psychiatric Nurses Association, & National Association of Psychiatric Health Systems, 2007). For example, say to the patient, "I notice that you are pacing up and down the hallway and that your fists are clenched." This gives the patient an opening to talk out the issues causing this behavior. Encouraging the patient to verbalize any issues decreases anxiety and tension and reduces the risk of escalation.

> ✓ **NOTE** Behavior in itself is a form of communication. When people feel agitated, their body language will reflect this. Being able to observe and interpret body language gives caregivers a window of opportunity for early intervention and successful de-escalation.

ASSESSING PATIENT BEHAVIOR FOR SIGNS OF AGITATION

Healthcare professionals must be able to assess the behavior of patients to detect signs of agitation (Lamont & Brunero, 2018). This involves asking patients what they are experiencing and how long any issues they are facing have existed. This helps you, the healthcare professional, determine exactly what the patients' present situation is, what (if any) problems are causing them distress, and whether the problem is temporary or permanent.

As you converse with the patients, you'll want to observe them closely. In particular, pay attention to the following:

- **The contents of the patients' responses.** What are they saying?

- **The patients' tone of voice.** Does their tone of voice make them seem angry or calm?

- **The patients' facial expression.** Are the patients smiling? Are they frowning? Are they expressionless?

- **The patients' demeanor.** Do the patients seem anxious, fearful, or calm?

- **The patients' hands.** Are the patients holding something? Are their hands hiding behind their back?

- **Whether anyone else is around.** Is anyone else involved in the issue at hand?

You must assess the situation to gain a full picture of what's going on. Only then can you determine what interventions are appropriate.

Anger: An Intense—and Often Misunderstood—Emotion

Anger is a normal human emotion. When someone feels ignored, misunderstood, or disrespected, they often feel angry (Boyd, 2008). This often occurs in mental health and other healthcare facilities.

Often, anger is expressed in a destructive way—aggressively or even violently (Gaynes et al., 2017). For example, those who are angry might threaten others or manipulate them in a way that is harmful (National Institute for Health and Clinical Excellence, 2005). Or, they might lash out verbally or physically. Often people who are angry feel cornered, which can result in its own set of aggressive behaviors (Boyd, 2008).

Interestingly, anger can sometimes be expressed in a positive way. For example, those suffering from substance abuse disorder could become so angry at their addiction, they decide to become clean and sober. Nurses can help patients express their anger in a positive way by encouraging them to talk things out rather than resorting to violence. Every time a nurse encourages a patient to do this, it decreases the risk of the patient ever becoming violent.

For information on de-escalating an angry patient, see Chapter 16, "De-Escalation of Angry Patients."

THE IMPORTANCE OF EARLY INTERVENTION

If a patient becomes agitated or aggressive, it's best to intervene right away. Research has shown that the earlier a de-escalation intervention is initiated, the better the chance of successful de-escalation (Richmond et al., 2012). Indeed, it is vital that healthcare staff intervene at the very first sign of escalation (Biancosino et al., 2009). It is much easier to de-escalate an individual who is mildly anxious or irritated than someone in a full-blown rage.

Intervening early can help break the cycle of escalation and prevent the patient from losing control (Littrell & Littrell, 1998). It also reduces the threat of injury to staff and patients. So, how early should you intervene? For best results, you should intervene at the first sign of agitation (Johnson & Delaney, 2007). That's not to say de-escalating later in the escalation cycle won't be effective. It might be. But it will take much longer for the agitated or aggressive person to achieve self-control.

> **? TIP** To enable early intervention, adequate acuity-based unit staffing is necessary.

REFERENCES

American Psychiatric Association, American Psychiatric Nurses Association, & National Association of Psychiatric Health Systems. (2007). *Learning from each other: Success stories and ideas for reducing restraint/seclusion in behavioral health*. Retrieved from http://www.restraintfreeworld.org/documents/Learning%20From%20Each%20Other.pdf

Biancosino, B., Delmonte, S., Grassi, L., Santone, G., Preti, A., Miglio, R., & De Girolamo, G. (2009). Violent behavior in acute psychiatric inpatient facilities: A national survey in Italy. *Journal of Nervous and Mental Disease, 197*(10), 772–782.

Boyd, M. A. (2008). *Psychiatric nursing: Contemporary practice* (4th ed.). Philadelphia, PA: Lippincott, Williams & Wilkins.

Byrnes , J. D. (2000) The aggression continuum: A paradigm shift. *Occupational Health & Safety, 69*(2), 70–71.

Caplan, G. (1964). *Principles of preventive psychiatry*. New York, NY: Basic Books, Inc.

Caplan, G. (1970). *The theory and practice of mental health consultation*. New York, NY: Basic Books, Inc.

Chabora, N., Judge-Gorny, M., & Grogan, K. (2003). The Four S Model in Action for de-escalation: An innovative state hospital-university collaborative endeavor. *Journal of Psychosocial Nursing and Mental Health Services, 41*(1), 22–28.

Cowin, L., Davies, R., Estall, G., Berlin, T., Fitzgerald, M., & Hoot, S. (2003). De-escalating aggression and violence in the mental health setting. *International Journal of Mental Health Nursing, 12*(1), 64–73.

Distasio, C. A. (1994). Violence in health care: Institutional strategies to cope with the phenomenon. *Health Care Supervisor, 12*(4), 1–34.

Gaynes, B. N., Brown, C. L., Lux, L. J., Brownley, K. A., Van Dorn, R. A., Edlund, M. J., … Lohr, K. N. (2017). Preventing and de-escalating aggressive behavior among adult psychiatric patients: A systemic review of the evidence. *Psychiatric Services, 68*(8), 819–831. doi: 10.1176/appi.ps.201600314

Hamrin, V., Iennaco, J., & Olsen, D. (2009). A review of ecological factors affecting inpatient psychiatric unit violence: Implications for relational and unit cultural improvements. *Issues in Mental Health Nursing, 30*(4), 214–226. doi: 10.1080/01612840802701083

Hilgers, J. (2003). Comforting a confused patient. *Nursing, 33*(1), 48–50.

Johnson, M. E., & Delaney, K. R. (2007). Keeping the unit safe: The anatomy of escalation. *Journal of the American Psychiatric Nurses Association, 13*(1), 42–50.

Lamont, S., & Brunero, S. (2018). The effect of a workplace violence training program for generalist nurses in the acute hospital setting: A quasi-experimental study. *Nurse Education Today, 68*, 45–52. doi: 10.1016/j.nedt.2018.05.008

Littrell, K. H., & Littrell, S. H. (1998). Current understanding of violence and aggression: Assessment and treatment. *Journal of Psychosocial Nursing and Mental Health Services, 36*(12), 18–24.

Lown, B. A., & Setnik, G. S. (2018). Utilizing compassion and collaboration to reduce violence in healthcare settings. *Israel Journal of Health Policy Research, 7*(1), 39. doi: 10.1186/s13584-018-0234-z

National Institute for Health and Clinical Excellence. (2005). Violence: The short-term management of disturbed/violent behaviour in in-patient psychiatric settings and emergency departments. *NICE Clinical Guidelines, No. 25* (pp. 19–81). London, UK: National Collaborating Centre for Nursing and Supportive Care.

Paterson, B., Leadbetter, D., & McComish, A. (1997). De-escalation in the management of aggression and violence. *Nursing Times, 93*(36), 58–61.

Richmond, J. S., Berlin, J. S., Fishkind, A. B., Holloman, G. H., Zeller, S. L., Wilson, M. P., … Ng, A. T. (2012). Verbal de-escalation of the agitated patient: Consensus statement of the American Association for Emergency Psychiatry Project BETA De-Escalation Workgroup. *Western Journal of Emergency Medicine, 13*(1), 17–25. doi: 10.5811/westjem.2011.9.6864

Simon, R. I., & Tardiff, K. (2008). *Textbook of violence assessment and management.* St. Louis, MO: American Psychiatric Publishing, Inc.

Tingleff, E. B., Bradley, S. K., Gildberg, F. A., Munksgaard, G., & Hounsgaard, L. (2017). "Treat me with respect." A systematic review and thematic analysis of psychiatric patients' reported perceptions of the situations associated with the process of coercion. *Journal of Psychiatric and Mental Health Nursing, 24*(9), 681–698. doi: 10.1111/jpm.12410

4

DE-ESCALATION TECHNIQUES

"Better than a thousand words, is one word that brings peace."
–Buddha

OBJECTIVES

- Discuss verbal de-escalation techniques

- Analyze distraction techniques

- Identify comfort measures

- Examine reality-orientation techniques

- Explore the relationship between stress and escalation

- Find out how to manage the environment to deal with aggressive behaviors

- Explore general principles for de-escalation

- Learn how to debrief, report, and document a de-escalation encounter

- Describe skills for working with families and caregivers

In today's stressful world, with its many conflicts and constant tension, it is imperative for all healthcare workers to know and use de-escalation techniques (Harwood, 2017; Hext, Clark, & Xyrichis, 2018). At any time, a healthcare worker could encounter an agitated person in the healthcare environment or in a professional role. How that healthcare worker responds can make the difference between whether the situation is peacefully resolved or whether it escalates to the level of physical aggression or violence toward others.

Psychological de-escalation techniques are among the most valuable skills a nurse or healthcare worker can possess. *De-escalation* is the process of helping a person regain self-control by using therapeutic communication and interventions to lower emotional tension, defuse the situation, and provide alternatives to escalation (Cowin et al., 2003; Distasio, 1994; Hamrin, Iennaco, & Olsen, 2009; Price & Baker, 2012). De-escalation is the least restrictive nonpharmacologic technique to prevent violence in a healthcare setting (Hext et al., 2018).

This chapter discusses key psychological de-escalation techniques. These include verbal, distraction, comfort, reorienting, and stress-management techniques, as well as milieu management. It also discusses principles and tips for safe and effective de-escalation. All nurses and healthcare workers need these vital skills to ensure a safe healthcare environment. Finally, the chapter discusses working with family members and caregivers and offers tips for handling an assortment of difficult situations.

VERBAL TECHNIQUES FOR DE-ESCALATION

The most important de-escalation technique is verbal de-escalation. Verbal de-escalation is both the simplest de-escalation technique and the easiest one to apply. *Verbal de-escalation* involves encouraging the agitated person to verbalize thoughts, feelings, and problems (Hallett & Dickens, 2015; Richmond et al., 2012). At the heart of verbal de-escalation is getting another person to talk.

> ✅ **NOTE** Verbal de-escalation is not about the nurse talking. It is about the nurse encouraging the agitated person to verbalize problems.

There are two purposes for verbal de-escalation. One is to assess the situation to identify what has led to the person's agitated behavior. This means asking the person questions to explore and understand the situation (Distasio, 1994). The other purpose is to help calm the person down. Research indicates that verbalizing one's problems can lead to calming and emotional healing (Freud, 1961; Shah et al., 2016). Encouraging people to verbalize their fears, anxiety, or anger instead of acting out those feelings is a vital part of the helping process.

> ✅ **NOTE** As you assess the situation, it's critical that you identify precipitating factors, antecedents, and triggers underlying the patient's behavior. Chapter 3, "Assessing an Escalating Situation for Early Intervention," discusses this in more detail.

Sigmund Freud (1961) developed the concept of the "talking cure" to promote emotional healing through verbalization. Freud (1961) found that when people talk about troubling personal issues, they begin to realize how to work out their problems themselves. Realization dawns when verbalization places the issue out in the open, releasing pent-up tension and anxiety, and promoting resolution. Verbal de-escalation is encouraging the person to speak, promoting calming as well as helping to restore self-control and balance.

> ✅ **NOTE** In mental health, this type of verbalization is called *ventilation*. It is similar to letting the air out of a balloon. When agitated individuals begin talking out problems, it takes some of the pressure off, causing de-escalation and defusing anger. Verbalization ventilates the anger and has a calming effect.

One of the most effective techniques to encourage verbalization—indeed, for any form of therapeutic communication—is to ask open-ended questions (Peplau, 1989). (Therapeutic communication is discussed in more detail in Chapter 5, "Therapeutic Communication for De-Escalation.") An open-ended question is one that cannot be answered with a yes or a no. Open-ended questions encourage the person to verbalize the issues that are causing internal turmoil. Examples of open-ended questions include, "What is upsetting you?" and, "What happened?" These simple phrases provide an opportunity for the person to talk out their problems, release tension, and decrease anxiety. This helps defuse the person's anger (Cowin et al., 2003).

> ✅ **NOTE** Encouraging those who are agitated to verbalize their emotions can help them develop anger-management skills. This can help prevent them from acting violently in the future (Maier, 1996).

Of course, it's not enough to simply ask questions. You must also listen to the patients' answers—or anything else they want to talk about. As they speak, give them your undivided attention. Show that you are listening by responding appropriately, whether verbally or nonverbally. This will help to keep them engaged (Hamrin et al., 2009; Karp, 2002). Also, don't rush them. Give them time to gather and communicate their thoughts. Rushing individuals will only escalate their aggressive behavior.

Avoid arguing with people. If they try to challenge you or shout obscenities, simply reply with a polite nod. Don't get defensive or engage in a power struggle. This helps set limits and prevents manipulative behavior on the part of the patients. Instead, simply redirect the conversation.

> ✅ **NOTE** Don't let the person push your buttons!

Maybe the patients don't want to talk to you. That's OK. In that case, you can encourage them to communicate with a friend or family member. This can help them calm down and achieve healing.

DISTRACTION FOR DE-ESCALATION

When faced with an agitated individual, distraction can be an effective de-escalation technique. This technique involves encouraging diversional activities to redirect the person, such as the following:

- **Working on a puzzle or playing a game.** If your facility has puzzles or games on hand, offer one to the agitated person. Or, ask a family member to bring one in from home.

- **Reading.** Reading a magazine, book, or spiritual text, such as a Bible, Koran, or similar text (depending on the person's faith), can be especially calming.

- **Watching TV or listening to music.** This can divert the person's attention from the upsetting issue.

- **Hands-on exercises.** Performing hand exercises or even just folding washcloths or towels can help some agitated people achieve a calm state—especially those who suffer from Alzheimer's or dementia.

- **Taking a short nap.** This can help the person re-center and regain self-control.

- **Drawing a picture.** The motion of the hand moving to draw can be both calming and comforting (American Psychiatric Association [APA], American Psychiatric Nurses Association, & National Association of Psychiatric Health Systems, 2007).

> ☑ **NOTE** Diversional activities are particularly calming for people who feel agitated due to boredom.

Reminiscence therapy is another beneficial diversional de-escalation technique to decrease anger and foster calm. *Reminiscence therapy* involves asking individuals to remember a pleasant event in the past, such as their wedding day or the day of the birth of their first grandchild. Often, when people reminisce in this way, they will also recall behaving appropriately during the event and begin to calm down (Oh, Fong, Hshieh, & Inouye, 2017). Reminiscence therapy is a particularly good de-escalation technique for patients with Alzheimer's or dementia (Seaward, 2012). In addition to calming the patients down, it helps improve their ability to remember the event (Cheong, 2004; Kneisl & Trigoboff, 2009).

CALMING COMFORT MEASURES

Some individuals with communication difficulties are unable to voice issues or needs and may display irritable or agitated behavior due to discomfort. For these individuals, offering a comfort measure may help de-escalate the situation (Hext et al., 2018). Here are several examples of calming comfort measures:

- **Offering a warm blanket.** Some individuals become agitated due to cold. Covering the patient with a warm blanket will defuse the anger caused by the patient's physical discomfort. You can also adjust the room temperature to provide warmth. Being warm may help the person settle down.

- **Massaging the patient's back.** This human touch can be healing, comforting, and calming—particularly for anxious Alzheimer's or dementia patients. Before giving a back massage, always ask for (and receive) permission. This conveys respect and trust, which is essential for de-escalation (Tingleff, Bradley, Gildberg, Munksgaard, & Hounsgaard, 2017).

- **Removing the patient from a chaotic environment.** Noisy and chaotic environments can be overwhelming for some patients and cause them to act out. This is especially true of patients with mental illness such as bipolar disorder and dementia. If an individual becomes agitated in a chaotic or noisy environment, placing this person in a quiet area may de-escalate the situation (Johnson & Hauser, 2001; Lancioni, Cuvo, & O'Reilly, 2002).

- **Taking the patient for a walk.** Going for a walk to enjoy the beauty of nature can be very calming. Even a walk around the unit is beneficial. The walk may also aid by simply removing the patient from more chaotic surroundings. The change of scenery and environment promotes comfort and harmony with others (Johnson & Hauser, 2001; Lancioni et al., 2002).

- **Offering a meal, snack, or beverage.** It may be that the agitated person is hungry or thirsty but unable to voice that need. For example, the patient may have missed a lunch tray or arrived at the facility before having had a chance to eat. Offering a meal, snack, or beverage can help a person who feels irritable or uncomfortable due to hunger to calm down. It also demonstrates caring and promotes therapeutic rapport with the caregiver.

> ☑ **NOTE** Comfort measures are particularly effective for calming the confused, the agitated, or those with impaired verbalization skills.

REORIENTING THE PATIENT TO REALITY

People suffering from altered perceptions or paranoid delusions due to conditions such as schizophrenia or dementia often become confused, agitated, or fearful that others want to harm them. Reorienting such individuals by informing them of the current date, time, place, and situation is an excellent de-escalation technique. It is also helpful to reassure such patients that they are in a safe place and that no one will harm them. Reorienting and reassuring the person in this way can help calm them (Duxbury & Whittington, 2005; Kneisl & Trigoboff, 2009).

DE-STRESS TO DE-ESCALATE

Stress is a primary trigger for agitation. Indeed, stress can quickly cause a person to become angry or even aggressive toward others. Teaching and encouraging the use of relaxation exercises that aid in reducing stress is an effective de-escalation technique. Exercises like diaphragmatic breathing, mental imagery, meditation, yoga, and progressive muscular relaxation can help individuals calm themselves and regain self-control (Seaward, 2012). Chapter 6, "Stress-Management Techniques," covers these exercises in more detail.

Another stress-relieving activity that can help de-escalate tense situations is journal writing. Writing in a journal helps people assess themselves, express themselves, and release their emotions, which in turn promotes self-control. The simple motion of the hand while writing is also soothing and comforting.

Finally, listening to music can help to alleviate stress (APA et al., 2007; Chabora, Judge-Gorny, & Grogan, 2003; Hilgers, 2003). In fact, music is one of the best techniques for de-escalation. Like the old idiom says, "Music can soothe the savage beast." When faced with an agitated patient, playing music with a slow tempo and no words works best. (Words tend to build anxiety and tension—especially the words in some of the music of today.) Or, just select something you know the person prefers.

> ☑ **NOTE** For more information about techniques to relieve patient stress, see Chapter 6.

MILIEU MANAGEMENT

An important component of effective de-escalation is milieu management. The *therapeutic milieu* is defined as the environment that surrounds a patient (Boyd, 2008). So, milieu management is about managing that environment.

The environment in which people find themselves greatly affects their behavior and interactions. Indeed, research indicates that environment is the most common reason for inpatient violence (Distasio, 1994). Overstimulation is a particular problem for some patients—particularly those who suffer from conditions such as bipolar and dementia. For these patients, overstimulation can drive agitation and aggression.

If a patient becomes overstimulated due to the environment, you'll need to minimize or eliminate certain environmental stimuli. One such stimulant is loud noise. Noise can trigger agitation in patients (Rueve & Welton, 2008). Reducing or eliminating loud noise or moving the patient to a less noisy or crowded area is an effective milieu-management intervention (Johnson & Hauser, 2001). A quiet environment is essential for fostering a safe therapeutic healthcare unit.

Harsh lighting can also irritate patients. So, dimming the lights is an excellent milieu-management intervention for patients who have normal vision and gait. Dim lighting is both calming and gentler on the eyes. After you dim the lights, encourage the patient to perform deep-breathing exercises or other relaxation techniques to reduce agitation (Caplan, 1964; Lancioni et al., 2002).

Beyond addressing noise and lighting issues, milieu management simply means minimizing general chaos and commotion.

> ✅ **NOTE** Milieu management doesn't just help de-escalate patients. Providing a calm therapeutic environment can prevent them from becoming aggressive in the first place.

PRINCIPLES OF SAFE AND EFFECTIVE DE-ESCALATION

Regardless of which de-escalation technique you use, there are several key principles for safe and effective de-escalation. These principles are as follows (Caroll, 2004):

- **Stay calm.** When approaching an agitated person with the intention to de-escalate, maintain a calm, caring, and professional demeanor—even if the patient challenges or insults you (Cowin et al., 2003; Price, Baker, Bee, & Lovell, 2018). In any tense situation, you as a nurse are a role model. If the person senses you are losing control, the situation will only worsen. You *must* stay calm and maintain your self-control to enable the person to retain self-control. By remaining calm and composed, you inspire others to do the same.

- **Remove the audience.** In the case of an inpatient mental health unit, if the patient acts out while onlookers are present—especially if the onlookers are peers of the verbally escalating individual—it tends to make the situation worse. Onlookers might themselves become agitators, encouraging the person to act out more violently. Or, the presence of onlookers might make it more difficult for the person to back down for fear of "losing face." So, when a patient acts out, you should remove the audience. You'll find it easier to de-escalate effectively in a one-on-one interaction with the patient than in a group setting with an audience of peers. Often, people act aggressively in front of others but back down when alone.

> ✅ **NOTE** In any tense encounter, helping the patient save face will prove beneficial (Edward, Giandinoto, Weiland, Hutton, & Reel, 2018).

- **Show respect.** Research has shown that one main reason people behave aggressively is that they feel they have been disrespected in some way (Johnson & Delaney, 2007; Tingleff et al., 2017). Research has also shown that showing respect to someone greatly reduces the likelihood that person will become aggressive (Juliana et al., 1997). Demonstrating respect in speech and manner can greatly reduce the risk of physical aggression.

- **Be mindful of your body language.** Often, as people become more agitated, they focus less on your words and more on your body language. For this reason, you should be mindful of what your body language conveys. Consider your demeanor, facial expression, posture, gestures, and movement. Also, be sure your body language matches your words. All this can help you avoid upsetting patients unnecessarily as well as communicate your support for them nonverbally.

- **Keep things short and simple.** When people are agitated, they perceive and process less information than when they are in a calm state. To avoid overwhelming an agitated person—which could increase anxiety and frustration and lead to further escalation—keep all communications, including directions, short, simple, clear, concise, and direct. A good rule of thumb is to use words that contain five or fewer letters and sentences with five or fewer words. Also avoid using slang, jargon, and colloquialisms.

- **Use proper paraverbals.** *Paraverbals* refers to the tone or pitch of the voice, the volume of the voice, the rate or rhythm of speech, gestures, and facial expressions. Using proper, or congruent, paraverbals enhances your chances of a successful de-escalation. In other words, your paraverbals must match your words, as identical statements can have completely opposite meanings depending on what paraverbals you use (Caroll, 2004). Using congruent paraverbals can help reduce the anxiety and tension that often precede dangerous behavior. This assists in calming the individual and restoring a sense of self-control.

- **Set limits.** The best way to set limits is to be nonconfrontational and respectful (Harwood, 2017; Roberton, Daffern, Thomas, & Martin, 2012). Don't overdo it, though. Set limits only as needed to protect the agitated person or others. And don't set a limit that you can't (or won't) enforce.

When setting limits, use language that is clear, specific, and direct. Explain the limit and the consequence of overstepping it (Kneisl & Trigoboff, 2009). Keep expectations reasonable and feasible. Avoid "personalizing" the limit. The idea is to show your acceptance of the person while rejecting the inappropriate behavior. This helps to protect the person's self-esteem while still enforcing behavioral limits. On a related note, try to provide opportunities for success. And when the person behaves within the limits you have set, acknowledge this to promote further compliance.

- **Offer choices.** Patients often feel powerless. This may cause them to act out in an attempt to wrest some control over their care and their lives (DelBel, 2003). One way you can help these frustrated patients is by offering two choices during a de-escalation intervention. For example, you might say, "Would you prefer for me to turn on the television or bring you a book to read?" Or you can negotiate and compromise with patients to develop new and better options. This empowers the patients—helping to restore their self-esteem and self-respect—while also enabling them to save face in the encounter.

> ✅ **NOTE** Sometimes it is not the de-escalation intervention that matters, but the fact that the patient was allowed to *choose* the de-escalation intervention.

- **Hold patients accountable for aggressive or violent behavior.** Call out patients when they act in an aggressive manner—but do it gently, and in such a way that you criticize the *behavior* rather than criticizing the patients. This way, the patients do not perceive the criticism as a personal attack. For example, say, "Your behavior of shouting loudly in the hallway is unnecessary and is frightening to everyone." Remind patients that they are partners in maintaining an environment that is safe for everyone, and that aggression and violence are not acceptable. Be aware, too, that some patients are desensitized to violence, often due to lifelong exposure to it. These patients may not even realize that violence is wrong. Explain to them that it is and that it will not be tolerated.

- **Be consistent.** Don't ignore patients' poor behavior one day and then call them out on it the next. On a related note, try to maintain consistency in inpatient unit routines and in staffing to reduce anxiety among patients.

- **Don't judge.** Maintaining a nonjudgmental attitude is essential for effective de-escalation. When patients are in crisis, it is *not* the time to judge, sermonize, criticize, or lecture them. Instead, partner with the patients to address their distress. This is particularly important for mentally ill and mentally challenged patients. Because these conditions are frequently stigmatized, patients who suffer from them face judgment by members of the community. They don't need it from you, too.

- **Give positive reinforcement.** Acknowledge when patients exhibit appropriate behavior. For example, say, "I am so proud of you for staying calm during that tense situation!" This will inspire the patient to continue to behave appropriately in the future.

- **Take a team approach.** It used to be that nurses were responsible for de-escalating their own patients. These days, de-escalation is a team effort. Whichever nurse has the best rapport with the agitated patient and is in the right frame of mind to take on the task is the one who should initiate de-escalation (Grover, 2005; Snorrason & Biering, 2018).

- **See it through.** De-escalation efforts should continue until patients completely regain self-control.

Tag-Teaming De-Escalation Duties

Like anyone, nurses have good and bad days. When nurses are having a bad day, they are not good candidates to de-escalate an agitated person—especially if that person is contributing to the bad day. In fact, nurses' own agitation might actually make things worse. Calm people *always* have the best chance of successfully de-escalating a patient.

Suppose Suzanne, the night nurse, receives a call. When she enters the patient's room, he throws urine in her face. Will this nurse be able to successfully de-escalate this patient? Well, the answer is no! In this case, a coworker should step in to de-escalate. In fact, that coworker should go one step further and take on the patient for the rest of the shift. Supporting and helping each other—it's what we healthcare professionals do.

TEST YOURSELF

DEALING WITH ESCALATING BEHAVIORS George is a 42-year-old patient on an inpatient unit. Lately he has become more aggressive toward staff and other patients. He constantly paces in the hall and mutters to himself. When approached by the nursing staff, he shouts and curses at them, saying, "You all are plotting against me!" The nurse recognizes these behaviors as indicators of escalation of aggressive behavior.

How would you handle this situation?

REFERENCES

American Psychiatric Association, American Psychiatric Nurses Association, & National Association of Psychiatric Health Systems. (2007). *Learning from each other: Success stories and ideas for reducing restraint/seclusion in behavioral health*. Retrieved from http://www.restraintfreeworld.org/documents/Learning%20From%20Each%20Other.pdf

Boyd, M. A. (2008). *Psychiatric nursing: Contemporary practice* (4th ed.). Philadelphia, PA: Lippincott, Williams & Wilkins.

Caplan, G. (1964). *Principles of preventive psychiatry*. New York, NY: Basic Books, Inc.

Caroll, V. (2004). Preventing violence in the healthcare workplace, *The Alabama Nurse, 31*(1), 23.

Chabora, N., Judge-Gorny, M., & Grogan, K. (2003). The Four S Model in Action for de-escalation: An innovative state hospital-university collaborative endeavor. *Journal of Psychosocial Nursing and Mental Health Services, 41*(1), 22–28.

Cheong, J. A. (2004). An evidence-based approach to the management of agitation in the geriatric patient. *Focus, 2*(2), 197–205.

Cowin, L., Davies, R., Estall, G., Berlin, T., Fitzgerald, M., & Hoot, S. (2003). De-escalating aggression and violence in the mental health setting. *International Journal of Mental Health Nursing, 12*(1), 64–73.

DelBel, J. C. (2003). De-escalating workplace aggression. *Nursing Management, 34*(9), 30–34.

Distasio, C. A. (1994). Violence in health care: Institutional strategies to cope with the phenomenon. *Health Care Supervisor, 12*(4), 1–34.

Duxbury, J., & Whittington, R. (2005). Causes and management of patient aggression and violence: Staff and patient perspectives. *Journal of Advanced Nursing, 50*(5), 469–478.

Edward, K. L., Giandinoto, J. A., Weiland, T. J., Hutton, J., & Reel, S. (2018). Brief interventions to de-escalate disturbances in emergency departments. *British Journal of Nursing, 27*(6), 322–327.

Freud, S. (1961). *The ego and the id*. In J. Strachey (Ed. and Trans.) *The standard edition of the complete psychological works of Sigmund Freud* (vol.19, pp. 3–66). London, UK: Hogarth Press.

Grover, S. (2005). Shaping effective communication skills and therapeutic relationships at work: The foundation of communication. *AAOHN Journal, 53*(4), 177–182.

Hallett, N., & Dickens, G. L. (2015). De-escalation: A survey of clinical staff in a secure mental health inpatient service. *International Journal of Mental Health Nursing, 24*(4), 324–333. doi: 10.1111/inm.12136

Hamrin, V., Iennaco, J., & Olsen, D. (2009). A review of ecological factors affecting inpatient psychiatric unit violence: Implications for relational and unit cultural improvements. *Issues in Mental Health Nursing, 30*(4), 214–226. doi: 10.1080/01612840802701083

Harwood, R. H. (2017). How to deal with violent and aggressive patients in acute medical settings. *The Journal of the Royal College of Physicians of Edinburgh, 47*(2), 94–101. doi: 10.4997/JRCPE.2017.218

Hext, G., Clark, L. L., & Xyrichis, A. (2018). Reducing restrictive practice in adult services: Not only an issue for mental health professions. *British Journal of Nursing, 27*(9), 479–485. doi: 10.12968/bjon.2018.27.9.479

Hilgers, J. (2003). Comforting a confused patient. *Nursing, 33*(1), 48–50.

Johnson, M. E., & Delaney, K. R. (2007). Keeping the unit safe: The anatomy of escalation. *Journal of the American Psychiatric Nurses Association, 13*(1), 42–50.

Johnson, M. E., & Hauser, P. M. (2001). The practices of expert psychiatric nurses: Accompanying the patient to a calmer personal space. *Issues in Mental Health Nursing, 22*(7), 651–668.

Juliana, C. A., Orehowsky, S., Smith-Regojo, P., Sikora, S. M., Smith, P. A., Stein, D. K., … Wolf, Z. R. (1997). Interventions used by staff to manage "difficult" patients. *Holistic Nursing Practice, 11*(4), 1–26.

Karp, S. J. (2002, Summer/Fall). Coercive tactics are no longer viable treatment methods. *Networks,* 13–15. Retrieved from http://www.restraintfreeworld.org/documents/Eliminating%20S&R.pdf

Kneisl, C. R., & Trigoboff, E. (2009). *Contemporary psychiatric-mental health nursing* (2nd ed.). Upper Saddle River, NJ: Prentice Hall.

Lancioni, G. E., Cuvo, A. J., & O'Reilly, M. F. (2002). Snoezelen: An overview of research with people with developmental disabilities and dementia. *Disability and Rehabilitation, 24*(4), 175–184.

Maier, G. J. (1996). Managing threatening behavior: The role of talk down and talk up. *Journal of Psychosocial Nursing and Mental Health Services, 34*(6), 25–30.

Oh, E. S., Fong, T. G., Hshieh, T. T., & Inouye, S. K. (2017). Delirium in older persons: Advances in diagnosis and treatment, *JAMA, 318*(12), 1,161–1,174. doi: 10.1001/jama.2017.12067

Peplau, H. (1989). *Interpersonal theory in nursing practice: Selected works of Hildegard E. Peplau.* New York, NY: Springer Publishing Company.

Price, O., & Baker, J. (2012). Key components of de-escalation techniques: A thematic synthesis. *International Journal of Mental Health Nursing, 21*(4), 309–310. doi: 10.1111/j.1447-0349.2011.00793.x

Price, O., Baker, J., Bee, P., & Lovell, K. (2018). The support-control continuum: An investigation of staff perspectives on factors influencing the success or failure of de-escalation techniques for the management of violence and aggression in mental health settings. *International Journal of Nursing Studies, 77,* 197–206. doi: 10.1016/j.ijnurstu.2017.10.002

Richmond, J. S., Berlin, J. S., Fishkind, A. B., Holloman, G. H., Zeller, S. L., Wilson, M. P., … Ng, A. T. (2012). Verbal de-escalation of the agitated patient: Consensus statement of the American Association for Emergency Psychiatry Project BETA De-Escalation Workgroup. *Western Journal of Emergency Medicine, 13*(1), 17–25. doi: 10.5811/westjem.2011.9.6864

Roberton, T., Daffern, M., Thomas, S., & Martin, T. (2012). De-Escalation and limit-setting in forensic mental health units. *Journal of Forensic Nursing, 8*(2), 94–101. doi: 10.1111/j.1939-3938.2011.01125.x

Rueve, M. E., & Welton, R. S. (2008). Violence and mental illness. *Psychiatry, 5*(5), 34–48.

Seaward, B. L. (2012). *Managing stress: Principles and strategies for health and well-being* (7th ed.). Burlington, VT: Jones & Bartlett Learning.

Shah, L., Annamalai, J., Aye, S. N., Xie, H., Pavadai, S. S., Ng, W., … Manickam, M. (2016). Key components and strategies utilized by nurses for de-escalation of aggression in psychiatric in-patients: A systemic review protocol. *JBI Database of Systemic Reviews and Implementation Reports, 14*(12), 109–118. doi: 10.11124/JBISRIR-2016-003219

Snorrason, J., & Biering, P. (2018). The attributes of successful de-escalation and restraint teams. *International Journal of Mental Health Nursing, 27*(6), 1,842–1,850. doi: 10.1111/inm.12493

Tingleff, E. B., Bradley, S. K., Gildberg, F. A., Munksgaard, G., & Hounsgaard, L. (2017). "Treat me with respect." A systematic review and thematic analysis of psychiatric patients' reported perceptions of the situations associated with the process of coercion. *Journal of Psychiatric and Mental Health Nursing, 24*(9), 681–698. doi: 10.1111/jpm.12410

5

THERAPEUTIC COMMUNICATION FOR DE-ESCALATION

"If you want peace, you don't talk to your friends. You talk to your enemies."

–Desmond Tutu

OBJECTIVES

- Explore the therapeutic communication cycle

- Distinguish between verbal and nonverbal communication

- Explore communication contexts

- Identify criteria for successful communication

- Explore fundamental elements of communication

- Discuss therapeutic communication techniques

- Explore ways to establish trust and therapeutic rapport

- Examine therapeutic interdisciplinary team communication

Noted psychiatrist Jurgen Ruesch proposed that communication could be defined as all processes by which one human being influences another (Kneisl & Trigoboff, 2009). He proposed further that communication is necessary for human survival. According to Ruesch, communication exists in many forms, both verbal and nonverbal. Communication is also one of the most difficult skills to master. It can take a lifetime of practice to perfect the skill of successful communication.

Therapeutic communication is defined more specifically as the set of communication techniques used by caregivers to focus on a patient's needs and to promote the continuous process of healing and change (Townsend, 2015).

Research indicates that therapeutic communication can reduce depressive symptoms and promote the emotional healing process (Curtis et al., 2016). Therapeutic communication can also foster increased insight and improved feelings of self-worth. Finally, therapeutic communication is *the* central element of the de-escalation techniques used to calm agitated patients and prevent violence (Lavelle et al., 2016). It uses holistic concepts of mental health, wellness, and recovery.

Therapeutic communication involves several key goals. One of these goals is to encourage verbalization to promote emotional equilibrium and inner peace. Another is to encourage problem-solving and enable decision-making for patient-centered care (Sheldon, 2005). Yet another is to facilitate a therapeutic nurse-patient relationship. This promotes optimal recovery outcomes.

THE THERAPEUTIC COMMUNICATION CYCLE

Research indicates that a significant number of inpatient violence incidents are triggered by poor communication skills among staff (Lanza, Kayne, Hicks, & Milner, 1991). The core of de-escalation training is developing good therapeutic communication skills to promote cooperation and avoid events that trigger violence. Using therapeutic communication skills can help nurses prevent patients from becoming agitated in the first place, thereby reducing the risk of inpatient violence.

Figure 5.1 illustrates the communication cycle. This cycle begins with an individual forming an idea. The idea is then "encoded," or placed into words, and transmitted in the form of a message to another person. This second person receives the message and interprets its content. The person then replies to the message with feedback, which prompts the formation of new ideas, thus beginning the cycle anew. This same cycle applies for therapeutic communication. The difference is that therapeutic communication specifically involves communicating in a respectful, gentle, and less provocative manner—in effect speaking to the patient using kindness, courtesy, and respect to prevent or defuse the escalation cycle. It is not so much what the nurse says as how the thoughts are communicated that defines therapeutic communication.

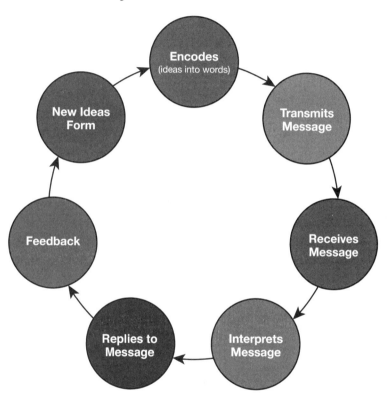

FIGURE 5.1 The therapeutic communication cycle.

VERBAL AND NONVERBAL COMMUNICATION

There are two main types of communication:

- **Verbal.** This refers to spoken-word, face-to-face communication. While most people tend to think of communication in primarily verbal terms, just 35% of communication is verbal in nature. (Note that written communication is essentially a transcript of verbal communication.)

■ **Nonverbal.** This refers to communication that doesn't involve the spoken word. It includes body language such as gestures, posture, and facial expressions; appearance; *proxemics* (the physical distance between people); and more. The majority of all human communication is nonverbal. In fact, research shows that nonverbal communication is the source of more than 65% of all messages received in a conversation (Hosley & Molle-Matthews, 2006).

> ☑ **NOTE** Communication refers not only to what words are spoken, but also to *how* they are spoken.

When communicating with an agitated or aggressive patient, you must remain aware of your body language (Hosley & Molle-Matthews, 2006). *Body language* is a type of nonverbal communication. It encompasses a range of behaviors, including behaviors relating to your voice; your head, eye, hand, and body movements; your facial expression; and your posture. But that's not all. How close or far you position yourself from the other person (called "proxemics") also transmits meaning. Maintaining a very close proximity can indicate anger, aggression, or a lack of respect, while staying too far away may indicate a feeling of distance or remove. Finally, your appearance sends a message—what clothes you wear, how you style your hair, whether you or your clothing appear tidy or unkempt, and so on. Figure 5.2 lists these forms of body language and provides examples of each.

Improving Nonverbal Communication

One way to improve communication generally is to work on your nonverbal communication. Here are a few tips:

■ **Be self-aware.** Pay attention to your body language, presence, and mannerisms. If you notice yourself exhibiting negative nonverbal behavior, you can work to change it.

■ **Relax.** The simple act of relaxing makes it easier for others to be relaxed in your presence.

■ **Use gestures judiciously.** If you use facial, hand, and body gestures too frequently, they may lose their effectiveness. Overdoing a gesture, such as constantly smiling or nodding your head, can appear insincere or simply become annoying to others.

■ **Practice.** Work on blending verbal messages with appropriate nonverbal cues such as hand gestures, posture, facial expression, and tone of voice. Do this in front of a mirror or ask for feedback from others to ensure you're communicating effectively.

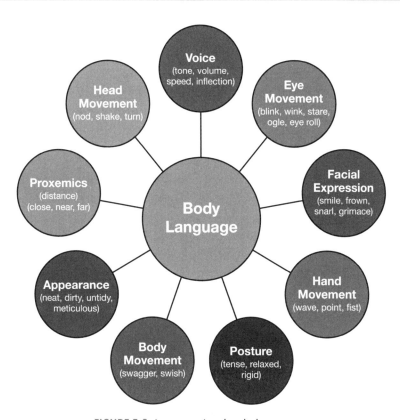

FIGURE 5.2 Interpreting body language.

COMMUNICATION CONTEXTS

Communication can occur in four different contexts:

■ **Interpersonal communication.** This is communication that involves two or more people. Effective interpersonal communication is vital to establishing the therapeutic alliance required for the successful de-escalation of agitation and aggression (Daffern, Day, & Cookson, 2012).

■ **Intrapersonal communication.** This describes communication with oneself—that is, one's internal dialogue (Kneisl & Trigoboff, 2009).

■ **Group communication.** This describes communication with a larger number of people who share a common interest.

■ **Societal communication.** This describes when a society or culture as a whole communicates a message to a designated individual or group.

CRITERIA FOR SUCCESSFUL COMMUNICATION

For communication to be successful, it must have a quality message. A successful communication also requires a recipient who is able to receive and interpret the message and to transmit a comprehendible reply.

Successful communication requires that four criteria be met. If these criteria are not met, communication is considered to be disturbed and cannot convey a comprehendible meaning. To ensure accurate, quality holistic care, nurses must meet these criteria in all communications. The criteria are as follows (Kneisl & Trigoboff, 2009):

■ **Efficiency.** This refers to your ability to effectively communicate your message in such a way that the recipient correctly interprets and understands it.

■ **Appropriateness.** This pertains to whether the message is being communicated at the proper time and in the proper context given the situation at hand.

■ **Flexibility.** This relates to whether the communication can be adapted for the message being communicated. A lack of flexibility means the message may be lost in an ever-changing healthcare environment.

■ **Feedback.** This describes the response from the individual who received the message. Feedback confirms not only the receipt of the message but also how the message was interpreted. When the recipient sends feedback, a sort of loop begins. Figure 5.3 illustrates this loop.

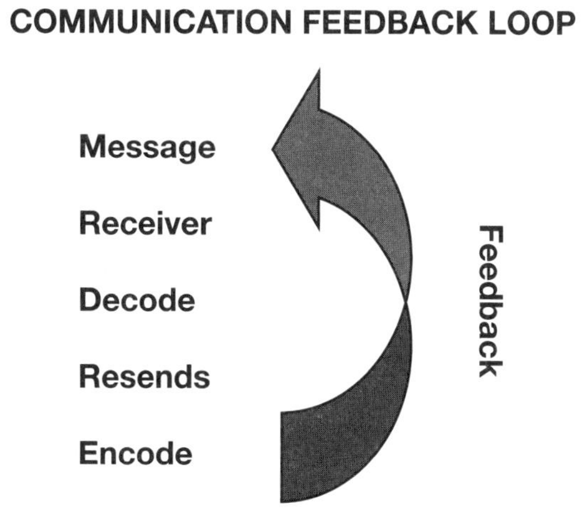

COMMUNICATION FEEDBACK LOOP

Message

Receiver

Decode

Resends

Encode

Feedback

FIGURE 5.3 The communication feedback loop.

FUNDAMENTAL ELEMENTS OF THERAPEUTIC COMMUNICATION

There are several fundamental elements of therapeutic communication (Hosley & Molle-Matthews, 2006):

- **Trust.** Trust is the basis of reliable communication. With trust, messages are heard and accepted as fact.

- **Empathy.** Empathy is your innate ability to understand what others are feeling and experiencing (Baile & Blatner, 2014). It's knowing how it feels to walk in someone else's shoes.

- **Respect.** Respect is the demonstration of consideration or esteem for another. Respect is vital to all therapeutic communication. It conveys trust in the therapeutic interaction. As mentioned in Chapter 4, "De-Escalation Techniques," research shows that the main reason people become physically aggressive is because they feel disrespected in some way (Johnson & Delaney, 2007; Tingleff, Bradley, Gildberg, Munksgaard, & Hounsgaard, 2017).

- **Congruence.** Congruence is when your nonverbal communications match your verbal messages—for example, smiling when you express something kind. This helps convey authenticity and genuineness. Congruence is an essential element of communication (Peplau, 1952). It helps ensure your communication is interpreted correctly.

- **Listening.** Listening is important to ensure complete comprehension. Show that you are listening by using verbal or nonverbal cues such as saying "OK" or nodding your head.

- **Self-awareness.** It's critical that when communicating a message, you remain aware of your facial expression and body language to ensure the message conveys what you intend it to. Self-awareness can allow for a truly therapeutic conversation—one in which all messages are received, heard, and understood (Northouse & Northouse, 1998).

> ✅ **NOTE** Many elements of therapeutic communication, such as trust, empathy, and respect, can be conveyed both verbally and nonverbally.

THERAPEUTIC COMMUNICATION TECHNIQUES

Therapeutic communication is a key component in de-escalation and for emotional healing. The goal of therapeutic communication is to encourage the patient to verbalize.

Simply offering one's self—sitting down and talking with the person about feelings—is an excellent therapeutic communication technique. Giving the person the chance to speak before issues become overwhelming reduces the chances of agitation (Juliana et al, 1997).

Using silence, presenting reality, focusing, summarizing, and giving feedback are other useful therapeutic communication techniques (Moosvi & Garbutt, 2018). Using silence gives the other person time to gather thoughts and to speak. Sometimes it even pushes an unwilling communicator to speak, just to fill the void. Presenting reality helps reorient the person back in the real world (necessary if the individual has altered perceptions of reality). Focusing enables you to draw out the main issues at hand. Summarizing the content of a communication can aid in understanding and future orientation (Hext, Clark, & Xyrichis, 2018; Hosley & Molle-Matthews, 2006). Receiving feedback from a communication ensures the intended meaning was conveyed.

Clarifying, imparting information, and problem-solving are yet more useful techniques. Clarifying involves helping the person voice concerns more clearly to ensure you understand them. Imparting information helps patients make educated decisions about their care. Finally, when you problem-solve, you aid the person in searching for viable alternatives related to health and optimal recovery outcomes. This allows for empowered decision-making.

As mentioned in Chapter 4, asking open-ended questions is essential in any therapeutic communication. Questions like, "What are you feeling?" or even, "How has your day been?" acknowledge the person, help you ascertain the situation, and offer a way to initiate conversation. Perception-checking is another key practice. This involves asking questions to ensure you understand the person—for example, "Do I understand this right—that you are upset because your cellphone is broken?" Repeating or paraphrasing the person's words is another way to achieve this, as well as to encourage further verbalization.

Chapter 4 also discussed *paraverbals*—the tone or pitch of your voice, the volume of your voice, the rate or rhythm of speech, your gestures and facial expressions, and so on. Successful therapeutic communication requires that you use paraverbals that are congruent with the content of your speech.

For effective therapeutic communication, keep these additional points in mind:

- **Focus on the patient.** The primary focus of every interaction should be the patient.

- **Maintain a professional attitude.** This helps to set the tone of the interaction. Be a professional in all therapeutic communication and duties.

- **Self-disclose with caution.** Only self-disclose with a specific therapeutic purpose in mind.

- **Maintain patient confidentiality.** Honor all HIPAA guidelines for privacy and patient rights (Stevenson, 1991).

- **Tailor your communication.** Assess the patient's intellectual level and communicate accordingly.

- **Combine theory with reality.** Use theory as a base from which to implement therapeutic interventions in reality (Stone, Singletary, & Richmond, 1999). For example, implement Peplau's interpersonal theory of therapeutic nurse patient interaction techniques by asking open-ended questions and encouraging patients to talk about themselves (1989).

- **Emphasize rationality.** Guide the patient to interpret experiences in a rational manner.

- **Use nonthreatening language.** Make observations about the patient like, "You look upset," and ask questions like, "Are you OK?"

- **Don't change the subject.** When the patient is communicating, avoid changing the subject unless doing so is needed for the patient's own well-being (Boyd, 2008).

- **Don't ask "why."** Often, patients don't know why they do what they do—particularly if they are mentally ill. In fact, that's probably why they're in treatment in the first place. Asking these patients "why" only reminds them of this and may cause them to feel even more frustrated or agitated than they did before. Instead, ask "what" or "how"—for example, "What happened to you?" This is more gentle and respectful.

- **Don't judge.** As mentioned in Chapter 4, when patients are in crisis, it is *not* the time to judge, sermonize, criticize, or lecture them. Instead, partner with patients to address their distress.

- **Inform, don't advise.** Nurses don't give advice. They provide information—giving patients the knowledge they need to make informed decisions on their own.

TEST YOURSELF

THERAPEUTIC COMMUNICATION Robert is a 27-year-old male inpatient who has been admitted to a medical facility for treatment of pancreatitis. Robert has a history of depression. He is isolative and withdrawn. Robert's facial expression is sad. He is frequently seen sitting alone in his room. Robert never has any visitors. Robert is visibly anxious and quiet.

What techniques would you use to interact with Robert to encourage therapeutic communication?

Therapeutic Communication With the Hard-of-Hearing

To be effective, therapeutic communication must be heard. To enable effective communication with the hard-of-hearing, keep these points in mind:

- **Move in close.** A distance of 3 to 6 feet from the patient works best.

- **Keep your face visible.** Place your face directly in front of the patient's to facilitate lip-reading (Kneisl & Trigoboff, 2009). Do not obscure your face with your hand, surgical mask, or other cover.

> ■ **Find out if the patient hears better in one ear than the other.** If one ear has better hearing, speak into that ear.
>
> ■ **Eliminate competing noise.** Turn off the TV or radio or move to a quieter environment (Jeffrey & Austen, 2005).
>
> ■ **Speak naturally.** Do not slow your speech.

TIPS TO ESTABLISH TRUST AND THERAPEUTIC RAPPORT

The goal during any de-escalation incident is to establish trust and develop therapeutic rapport. You want to partner with the patient to promote recovery. The following tips—in conjunction with the communication skills described in this chapter—are meant to help you do just that:

- **Knock.** Knock before entering a patient's room to show your respect.

- **Introduce yourself.** If this is your first time interacting with the agitated patient, introduce yourself by stating your name and position, and tell the patient why you are approaching. This will get the interaction off to a good start.

- **Address the patient by name or use an honorific.** Address the patient by name—for example, Mr. or Mrs. Smith. Or, use an honorific such as sir or ma'am unless given permission to use a more familiar form of address. This helps convey your respect for the patient.

- **Offer to help.** Tell the person that you are available to help, and ask what you can do to be of assistance. Simply offering to help someone conveys caring. It shows that you recognize the patient's needs and want to address them.

- **Problem-solve.** Ask the patient, "What can I do to help you right now?" Then offer to help the patient sort through the possible answers.

- **Be polite, courteous, and compassionate.** Show respect for the patient by being polite, courteous, and compassionate—while still remaining firm—in every interaction.

- **Show empathy.** Often, communicating empathy—demonstrating that you care and want to help—is enough to defuse a tense situation (Gaynes et al., 2017).

> ✅ **NOTE** Sometimes nurses have trouble expressing empathy to patients in a manner they can understand. One way to convey empathy is to begin a sentence with a phrase such as, "Because I am concerned about your well-being..." You can then go on to finish the sentence—for example, saying, "I want you to know I am available to sit down and speak with you at any time about what you are feeling."

- **Reassure the patient.** Inform the patient of personal safety. This simple statement reduces the risk of escalation due to ignorance or fear.

- **Model correct behavior.** Human beings naturally copy the behavior of others. So, when you exhibit correct behavior, your patients will often follow suit. In other words, when dealing with an agitated patient, remaining calm and composed will often cause the patient to behave in kind.

- **Speak calmly, slowly, and softly.** This will help defuse the situation.

- **Pause to encourage the person to talk.** Pausing gives the person time to gather and clarify thoughts. Pausing also gives the person an opportunity to take a breath and calm down.

- **Restate the patient's main point.** Using your own words, repeat back to the patient the main content of what's been communicated. That way you'll know you understood the patient correctly.

- **Reflect the patient's main emotional theme.** Ensure you understood the patient correctly by identifying and repeating back the main emotional theme of anything that's been communicated.

- **Focus the message.** Ask questions to help the patient focus on key concerns (Craven & Hirnle, 2009; Hosley & Molle-Matthews, 2006).

- **Engage in further questioning.** Encourage the patient to elaborate to ensure the problem at hand is described fully.

- **Don't change the subject.** When the patient is speaking, don't change the subject—unless doing so is necessary for the patient's well-being. Allow the patient to talk about anything for the ventilation of emotions.

- **Don't make promises you can't keep.** For example, do not promise the patient you will be back in the room in 15 minutes if you aren't sure you can be there on time.

- **Be honest.** Tell the patient the truth. For example, if you do not know for certain the patient's discharge date, say so. Then refer the patient to the physician or some other person who may be able to give an accurate time frame for discharge.

- **Apologize.** If your conversation with the patient reveals provocation by a staff member, apologize on behalf of the organization.

- **Don't take things personally.** Insults or derogatory comments made by the patient to healthcare staff in the heat of anger are usually not meant as personal attacks. Most likely, the patient's anger originates from her own personal issues or stressors.

- **Encourage the patient to regain self-control.** As you speak to the patient, convey that it is best to regain self-control (American Psychiatric Association, American Psychiatric Nurses Association, & National Association of Psychiatric Health Systems, 2007; Caplan, 1964; Gately & Stabb, 2005; Hilgers, 2003). That being said, don't encourage compliance by threatening negative consequences. Instead, communicate your positive expectations.

- **Identify strengths.** Then build on these strengths to help the patient regain self-control.

REFERENCES

American Psychiatric Association, American Psychiatric Nurses Association, & National Association of Psychiatric Health Systems. (2007). *Learning from each other: Success stories and ideas for reducing restraint/seclusion in behavioral health.* Retrieved from http://www.restraintfreeworld.org/documents/Learning%20From%20Each%20Other.pdf

Baile, W. F., & Blatner, A. (2014). Teaching communication skills: Using action methods to enhance role-play in problem-based learning. *Simulation in Healthcare, 9*(4), 220–227. doi: 10.1097/SIH.0000000000000019

Boyd, M. A. (2008). *Psychiatric nursing: Contemporary practice* (4th ed.). Philadelphia, PA: Lippincott, Williams & Wilkins.

Caplan, G. (1964). *Principles of preventive psychiatry.* New York, NY: Basic Books, Inc.

Craven, R. F., & Hirnle, C. J. (2009). *Fundamentals of nursing: Human health and function* (6th ed.). Philadelphia, PA: Lippincott Williams & Wilkins.

Curtis, J. R., Treece, P. D., Nielsen, E. L., Gold, J., Ciechanowski, P. S., Shannon, S. E., … Engelberg, R. A. (2016). Randomized trial of communication facilitators to reduce family distress and intensity of end-of-life care. *American Journal of Respiratory and Critical Care Medicine, 193*(2), 154–162. doi: 10.1164/rccm.201505-0900OC

Daffern, M., Day, A., & Cookson, A. (2012).Implications for the prevention of aggressive behavior within psychiatric hospitals drawn from interpersonal communication theory. *International Journal of Offender Therapy and Comparative Criminology, 56*(3), 401–419.

Gately, L. A., & Stabb, S. D. (2005). Psychology students' training in the management of potentially violent clients. *Professional Psychology: Research and Practice, 36*(6), 681–687.

Gaynes, B. N., Brown, C. L., Lux, L. J., Brownley, K. A., Van Dorn, R. A., Edlund, M. J., … Lohr, K. N. (2017). Preventing and de-escalating aggressive behavior among adult psychiatric patients: A systemic review of the evidence. *Psychiatric Services, 68*(8), 819–831.

Hext, G., Clark, L. L., & Xyrichis, A. (2018). Reducing restrictive practice in adult services: Not only an issue for mental health professions. *British Journal of Nursing, 27*(9), 479–485. doi: 10.12968/bjon.2018.27.9.479

Hilgers, J. (2003). Comforting a confused patient. *Nursing, 33*(1), 48–50.

Hosley, J., & Molle-Matthews, E. (2006). *A practical guide to therapeutic communication for healthcare professionals.* St. Louis, MO: Saunders.

Jeffrey, D., & Austen, S. (2005). Adapting de-escalation techniques with deaf service users. *Nursing Standard, 19*(49), 41–47. doi: 10.7748/ns2005.08.19.49.41.c3934

Johnson, M. E., & Delaney, K. R. (2007). Keeping the unit safe: The anatomy of escalation. *Journal of the American Psychiatric Nurses Association, 13*(1), 42–50.

Juliana, C. A., Orehowsky, S., Smith-Regojo, P., Sikora, S. M., Smith, P. A., Stein, D. K., … Wolf, Z. R. (1997). Interventions used by staff to manage "difficult" patients. *Holistic Nursing Practice, 11*(4), 1–26.

Kneisl, C. R., & Trigoboff, E. (2009). *Contemporary psychiatric-mental health nursing* (2nd ed.). Upper Saddle River, NJ: Prentice Hall.

Lanza, M. L., Kayne, H. L., Hicks, C., & Milner, J. (1991). Nursing staff characteristics related to patient assault. *Issues in Mental Health Nursing, 12*(3), 253–265.

Lavelle, M., Stewart, D., James, K., Richardson, M., Renwick, L., Brennan, G., & Bowers, L. (2016). Predictors of effective de-escalation in acute inpatient psychiatric settings. *Journal of Clinical Nursing, 25*(15–16), 2,180–2,188. doi: 10.1111/jocn.13239

Moosvi, K., & Garbutt, S. (2018). Shifting strategies: Using film to improve therapeutic communication and nursing education. *Nursing Education Perspectives.* doi:10.1097/01.NEP.00000000000000431

Northouse, P. G., & Northouse, L. J. (1998). *Health communications: Strategies for health professionals* (3rd ed.). Stanford, CT: Pearson.

Peplau, H. E. (1952). *Interpersonal relations in nursing: A conceptual frame of reference for psychodynamic nursing.* New York, NY: Putnam.

Peplau, H. E. (1989). *Interpersonal theory in nursing practice: Selected works of Hildegard E. Peplau.* New York, NY: Springer Publishing Company.

Sheldon, L. K. (2005). *Communication for nurses: Talking with patients.* Boston, MA: Jones & Bartlett Learning.

Stevenson, S. (1991). Heading off violence with verbal de-escalation. *Journal of Psychosocial Nursing and Mental Health Services, 29*(9), 6–10.

Stone, G., Singletary, M., & Richmond, V. P. (1999). *Clarifying communication theories: A hands-on approach.* New York, NY: John Wiley & Sons.

Tingleff, E. B., Bradley, S. K., Gildberg, F. A., Munksgaard, G., & Hounsgaard, L. (2017). "Treat me with respect." A systematic review and thematic analysis of psychiatric patients' reported perceptions of the situations associated with the process of coercion. *Journal of Psychiatric and Mental Health Nursing, 24*(9), 681–698. doi: 10.1111/jpm.12410

Townsend, M. C. (2015). *Psychiatric mental health nursing: Concepts of care in evidence-based practice* (8th ed.). Philadelphia, PA: F. A. Davis Company.

6

STRESS-MANAGEMENT
TECHNIQUES

"World peace begins with inner peace."
–Dalai Lama

O B J E C T I V E S

- Explain the stress response

- Identify types of stress

- Explore causes of stress

- Describe holistic stress management

- Learn how to perform diaphragmatic breathing

- Find out how to use mental imagery

- Learn the steps for meditation

- Discover the benefits of progressive muscular relaxation

Stress is one of the leading causes of anger, aggression, and violence. It's also a major contributing factor in depression and resultant suicide. Stress triggers negative emotions that increase the risk of danger to self or others. Stress research indicates that at least 20% of Americans experience high levels of hostile anger (Seaward, 2012).

Stress is a driving force of healthcare violence (The Joint Commission, 2018; Lown & Setnik, 2018). Stress is omnipresent in healthcare facilities. Patients experience stress from long waits, crowding, and fear of pain associated with invasive procedures and tests. They may also suffer from the stress of coping with a major or even life-threatening medical condition. This may cause patients to feel as though they are no longer able to cope. This may increase the risk of verbal or physical violence. This creates a significant risk for healthcare violence (Arnetz et al., 2015; Gillespie, Gates, Miller, & Howard, 2010; The Joint Commission, 2018).

Patients aren't the only ones who experience stress in a healthcare environment. Their family members also suffer from stress—for example, stress associated with caregiver responsibilities or grief. And nurses and other healthcare staff suffer from the stress associated with long hours of providing care—sometimes with only minor support in their duties from colleagues and interdisciplinary staff and little emotional support offered.

Healthcare environments are a toxic soup of stress-related triggers to aggression and violence. As stress mounts, the risk of healthcare violence rises. In one research study on healthcare violence, more than 36% of emergency department nurses reported being assaulted during the previous 12 months. Violence and stress are some of the major reasons nurses leave the workforce (International Council of Nurses, 2007). Educating nurses on stress management for self-care as well as how to educate patients and family members on these beneficial techniques is a formidable de-escalation intervention to prevent healthcare violence (Bronk, 2019).

THE FUNDAMENTAL ELEMENTS OF ALL HUMAN BEINGS

Psychologist Carl Jung (1964) once wrote, "Modern man is sick because he is not whole." I would argue that in fact, modern man is sick because he suffers from stress, and stress destroys holistic wellness.

All human beings are made up of many complex elements:

- **Our physical bodies.** We have physical bodies, but we are not just our physical bodies.

- **Emotions.** We can feel, recognize, and control our own emotions.

- **Intellect.** Our intellect or mental capacities enable us to perceive and know things and to communicate with each other.

- **Spirit.** As spiritual beings, we can develop higher levels of consciousness and sense a higher power greater than ourselves that gives meaning and purpose to our life.

Only when these elements are in balance are we truly whole. This is called *holistic wellness* (Fiandaca et al., 2017; Seaward, 2012). (See Figure 6.1.)

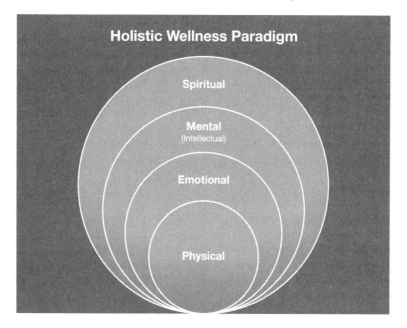

FIGURE 6.1 Holistic wellness paradigm.

Stress has a profound negative effect on holistic wellness. Indeed, research has revealed a connection between stress and both physical illness and psychological problems (Vinstrup, Jakobsen, Calatayud, Jay, & Andersen, 2018). Stress fuels depression and anger, which can lead to suicide or violence (Buhmann, Jungnickel, & Lehmann, 2018). Simply put, stress can be devastating to us as individuals and to our culture as a whole.

Stress-management techniques can help us reduce or eliminate stressful states. The primary goal of these techniques is to promote physical, emotional, mental, and spiritual health. This chapter discusses steps that anyone can take to reduce stress and to restore calm and homeostasis.

> ☑ **NOTE** Helping patients overcome stress is the single most important prevention and de-escalation intervention.

THE STRESS RESPONSE

The stress response is a primitive mechanism that our species developed to survive (Ketchesin, Stinnett, & Seasholtz, 2017). When ancient humans faced danger such as a predator, their stress response kicked in, which released a flood of hormones that either geared them up to fight for survival or gave them an extra jolt of speed to allow them to flee. This is called the "fight-or-flight response."

Few modern people find themselves chased by predators, but we still experience the stress response. Typically, this response is activated by a psychological stressor. For example, we might be sitting at our desk, fretting about an upcoming deadline, when the stress response hits. Suddenly, we are bombarded with epinephrine, catecholamine, and adrenal cortisol (Ketchesin et al., 2017). This hormonal flood makes our heart race, raises our blood pressure, accelerates our respiration, and gears up our body to fight or flee to survive (Yu et al., 2019). There's just one problem: We *can't* fight or flee. We must continue to sit at our desk while experiencing this overpowering stress response.

When people in the midst of the stress response cannot fight or flee, they cannot expend the hormonal flood. As a result, their body gets stuck in overdrive. But the human body is not made to withstand the fight-or-flight stress response for a prolonged period. This response is meant only for the short term. When this response lasts longer than it should, it burns people out both mentally and physically (Ketchesin et al., 2017). It weakens the body and opens it up to infection and disease (Seaward, 2012).

The six leading causes of death are coronary heart disease (CHD), cancer, lung ailments, accidents, cirrhosis of the liver, and suicide (Cohen, Edmondson, & Kronish, 2015; Esler, 2017). Stress is linked to all of these. CHD in particular is a lifestyle disease that is directly related to stress (Li & Goldsmith, 2012). Stress is also linked to conditions such as migraine headaches, female infertility, ulcers, common cold, insomnia, and hypertension (Yu et al., 2019). Stress can trigger practically anything from herpes to hemorrhoids. Stress also brings about an increase in alcoholism, drug addiction, self-mutilation, child and spouse abuse, suicide, and homicide.

> ☑ **NOTE** Research indicates that 70 to 80% of all incidences of disease are stress-related and that more than 50% of doctor visits are linked to stress. It's no wonder Americans spend more than $400 billion every year treating stress-related diseases (Ketchesin et al., 2017; Seaward, 2012).

TYPES OF STRESS

There are three types of stress:

- **Eustress.** Eustress is sometimes called positive stress. An example of an event that causes eustress might be starting at a new job. Eustress often feels exciting. It motivates us to perform at our best.

- **Neustress.** Neustress is neutral stress. Seaward defines neustress as "any kind of information or sensory stimulus that is perceived as unimportant or inconsequential" (2012, p. 9). You might experience neustress while watching a news report on a deadly earthquake on another continent. You feel sad about the news, but because you are not there, nor is anyone you know, it doesn't have much of an impact.

- **Distress.** This is defined as the negative interpretation of an event (real or imagined) that is deemed threatening and promotes continued feelings of fear or anger (Seaward, 2012). An example of an event that causes this type of distress might be the death of a spouse, loved one, or close friend. This is the kind of stress that you cannot shake off. When people speak about stress, this is generally the type they mean. Patients and family members of patients in healthcare facilities frequently experience this type of overwhelming stress.

Stress can be either acute or chronic (Seaward, 2012). *Acute stress* is high-intensity but lasts only for a short time. A person might experience acute stress while getting stopped for a traffic ticket. *Chronic stress* is low-intensity but prolonged. Financial problems are a common cause of chronic stress.

> ☑ **NOTE** The worst type of stress is chronic stress. The longer a person is under stress, the more devastating the effects. It's far better to experience acute stress than chronic stress.

COMMON CAUSES OF STRESS IN THE MODERN WORLD

Recent years have brought a dramatic increase in stress levels. Stressors in our modern world include financial problems—perhaps due to the recent economic recession (or fears of future meltdowns); unemployment (and the resultant financial stress of job loss); fears of global warming and dramatic weather conditions; and more. Illness or injury and a lack of insurance is another prominent stressor.

One major modern stressor pertains to the advent of communications technologies like computers, the internet, and cellphones. Modern technology was created to be a servant of humankind. But in many ways it has turned the tables on us. We have become the slaves of technology.

It used to be that people could take time to themselves to relax and recharge. There was a clear dividing line between employees' work life and their home life. Not anymore. Now, thanks to modern technology, we feel we must be available to others 24 hours a day, 7 days a week (Cohen et al., 2015). We bring our laptops home so we can work after hours and even on vacation. We don't give ourselves time to rest and revitalize. We burn the candle at both ends and in the middle, and we are getting burned with stress. Add to that other new stressors associated with technology—for example, protecting ourselves from bad actors like phishers, spammers, scammers, spoofers, and social media trolls—and it's no wonder we're all such a mess.

> ☑ **NOTE** There is a term for this type of stress: techno stress. *Techno stress* is stress associated with advancing technology that has brought about non-stop communication and stress without relief.

Speaking of stress at work, there's another reason for it: the rapid rate of technological change in the modern workplace. As soon as you become adept at using a piece of software or digital equipment, it is inevitably updated to a totally different system—meaning you have to start the learning process all over again. This endless cycle of technological change results in stress on top of stress.

And let's not forget the impact of all this technology on family dynamics. It used to be that people could escape family issues while they were at work or away from home. Not anymore. Thanks to the cellphone, we engage in family chaos, commotion, and crisis all day every day.

To make matters worse, the number of stressors in our lives appears to be increasing. Things aren't getting better; they're getting worse. Research indicates that millennials (born between the early 1980s and mid-1990s) and Generation X (born between the mid-1960s and early 1980s) report higher stress levels than any other generation, including baby boomers (born between 1946 and 1964). In addition, 44% of millennials and Generation Xers report irritability and anger from stress (American Psychological Association, 2012). At no other time has there been so much stress and so little peace.

> ☑ **NOTE** Different cultures view stress differently. Eastern cultures see stress as the absence of inner peace. In other words, stress originates from within. In contrast, Western cultures see stress as an inability to cope with a perceived (real or imagined) threat to an individual's physical, mental, emotional, or spiritual well-being (Seaward, 2012).

HOLISTIC STRESS MANAGEMENT

Holistic stress management involves integrating, balancing, and harmonizing all aspects of the body, emotions, intellect, and spirit to move from a place of fear to a place of love and compassion for the self and others (Yu et al., 2019). The secret to stress management is very simple: It is learning to live in the present moment. It is said that the sparrow does not worry about what tomorrow brings. We need to become more like the sparrow: to live our lives one day—one moment—at a time.

> ☑ **NOTE** Stress management is about balancing the ego with the soul— uniting the conscious and unconscious mind. It's about learning to live our lives in peace and harmony with ourselves and with others.

There are several effective techniques to help individuals reduce stressful states, restore calm, and find peace. These include (Smith, Hancock, Blake-Mortimer, & Eckert, 2007; Travis et al., 2018):

- **Diaphragmatic breathing.** This is a form of controlled deep breathing that is relaxing and helps promote peace and calm.

- **Meditation.** This practice involves emptying the mind of ego-based worries to induce a tranquil state.

- **Mental imagery.** This practice entails using your mind to visualize relaxing scenes, engaging in health-conscious behavior, enjoying success, or healing the body (Stefanaki et al., 2015).

- **Progressive muscular relaxation (PMR).** PMR is a progressive tensing and relaxing of muscle groups to promote physical relaxation. This practice is especially beneficial for reducing anger (Sahranavard, Esmaeili, Dastjerdi, & Salehiniya, 2018).

These four techniques are explored in more detail in this chapter.

Other practices for reducing stress include:

- **Aromatherapy.** This involves diffusing a pleasant scent throughout the environment to soothe and calm.

- **Comfort measures.** This could include giving the patient a back massage for calming purposes.

- **Yoga.** Yoga is a beneficial stress management technique. Yoga focuses on physical balance and breathing for the purposes of calming, comforting, and relaxing, as well as general stress relief.

- **Music therapy.** This involves listening to music that is pleasurable and relaxing. Music therapy is one of the easiest and best stress-management techniques.

- **Relaxation recordings.** Listening to relaxation recordings can be soothing and calming (Keane, 2006; Power, 2010).

- **Autogenic training.** Autogenics is self-regulation to promote human relaxation based on self-awareness. It involves sending messages to the body to promote relaxation. For example, a person might repeat to himself "my breathing is slow and relaxed" or "my breathing is calm and comfortable" six or eight times.

- **Physical exercise and a healthy diet.** This invigorates the body to reduce tension (Edwards & Loprinzi, 2018).

- **Reduction of stressors.** This involves making an effort to reduce tensions that cause overwhelming stress. For example, if problems with parenting are a source of stress, a person might seek to reduce this stressor by attending family counseling or even parenting classes. Or, if financial problems are a main source of stress, a person might attempt to reduce this stressor by increasing income or paying down debt. The idea is to eliminate as many stressors as possible and feasible for holistic mental health.

Stress-management techniques decrease tension and promote the relaxation response for health, wellness, and recovery.

> ☑ **NOTE** It all begins with you. Be good to yourself, and your stress will lessen.

DIAPHRAGMATIC BREATHING

Diaphragmatic breathing—also called controlled breathing, deep breathing, or primal breathing—is an effective stress-management technique. It involves breathing from the lower stomach or diaphragm rather than from the thoracic area.

Diaphragmatic breathing is the healthiest way to breathe. It increases oxygenation in body tissue (Yong, Lee, & Lee, 2018) and activates vital energy in the body. In yoga it is called *pranayama*, meaning the restoration of energy or life force (Li & Goldsmith, 2012). It is the "breath behind the breath"—the most healing and energizing way to breathe. Diaphragmatic breathing also decreases chronic pain.

> ☑ **NOTE** Diaphragmatic breathing is how infants breathe. Although we later learn how to breathe using our chest, we were all born belly-breathing, and we revert to belly-breathing when we sleep.

Diaphragmatic Breathing Steps

1. Loosen your garments, remove your watch and shoes, and sit or lie comfortably in a chair or on the floor.

2. Place one hand on your chest and the other on your stomach.

3. Slowly inhale deeply through your nose or mouth, breathing into your lower diaphragm. Visualize healing energy flowing into your body.

4. Pause and hold the breath for 15 to 30 seconds.

5. Slowly exhale. Visualize the air leaving your mouth as dark, cloudy smoke. This symbolizes the stress, frustration, toxins, tension, and anxiety leaving your body.

6. Pause and rest, and then repeat.

7. Continue the breathing exercise for 5 to 10 minutes or until your visualization of the exhalation is clear.

MENTAL IMAGERY

Guided mental imagery is an exercise in which an instructor, therapist, or counselor guides people through a series of visualizations to build a pleasant image in their mind. They then engage their senses to bring this pleasant image to life in their mind (Beizaee et al., 2018). Mental imagery can also be done alone by imagining a beautiful image in your mind of a pleasant daydream to escape to. Mental imagery forms a holistic connection of the body, emotions, intellect, and spirit. Mental imagery can help people overcome obstacles, attain goals, and improve their overall state of physical and mental health (Anagnostouli, Babili, Chrousos, Artemiadis, & Darviri, 2018).

Mental Imagery Origins

Mental imagery emerged as an ancient healing technique in virtually every culture. For example, it was used by Australian Aborigines, in American Indian cultures, by Hindu yogis, and by the ancient Greeks. But it was not until the 20th century that it began to be used in Western medicine. Freud and Jung introduced mental imagery into psychoanalysis during the early 1900s. And in the 1970s, Carl and Stephanie Simonton used mental imagery to relieve pain in cancer patients (Grossert et al., 2016). Their work kicked off research into the benefits of mental imagery in clinical health settings.

There are four main types of mental imagery (Beizaee et al., 2018):

- Scenes that are tranquil and comforting, to induce calm

- Scenes in which the individual is seen engaging in a health-conscious behavior, such as becoming clean and sober, to drive positive behavioral changes

- Scenes in which the individual enjoys success of some sort—for example, crossing the finish line at the end of a marathon

- Visualizations of damaged or diseased organs or tissue being healed, to promote health and physical recovery from illness

Guided Mental Imagery: Painted Sails

Here's an example of a guided imagery script to induce calm:

- Close your eyes and imagine you are sailing away in a beautiful sailboat with brightly painted red and blue sails. As the sailboat glides quietly on the swift ocean current, you toss all your worries, cares, and stress onto the banks of the retreating shore.

- Forgive

- Forgive

- As the sailboat skips lightly over the vividly blue sea and you watch the glimmering shoreline fade away in the distance, you feel all your stress, tension, and anxiety release and dissipate.

- The sea breeze ruffles your hair. You feel the warm sun on your face and taste the salt spray on your lips. As the boat glides lightly over the shimmering waves of the peaceful ocean's azure blue depths, you feel its soft motion at your feet.

- Overhead, brown pelicans fly in a sky of brilliant blue, as small fluffy white clouds drift across the face of the sun. Seagulls with sleek, white feathers swim into the ocean's translucent waves. In the distance, other sailboats with bright blue sails float lightly over the blue ocean surf. All is calm and relaxed. All is serene and comforting.

- As you glide along in the sailboat over the ocean waves, you breathe deeply of the clean, fresh, vitalizing sea air. With each deep breath, your body feels rejuvenated, strong, and revitalized with healing energy.

> - Inhale….(pause 5 seconds)…..Exhale
>
> - Inhale….(pause 5 seconds)…..Exhale
>
> - Inhale….(pause 5 seconds)…..Exhale
>
> - Inhale….(pause 5 seconds)…..Exhale
>
> - Beside the bow of the sailboat, you see three playful blue dolphins. The dolphins dance in the sailboat's wake, chasing the sea foam over the surf as the sailboat quietly sails away. All is peaceful and calm. All is peaceful and calm.

Mental imagery is an effective way to reduce stress, tension, and anxiety and to prevent or reduce agitation (Anagnostouli et al., 2018). But that's not all. It also promotes holistic wellness by providing other benefits. For example, it can:

- Relieve symptoms of depression and anxiety (Beizaee et al., 2018)

- Improve emotional regulation and mental health (Edwards, Rhodes, Mann, & Loprinzi, 2018)

- Aid in pain management

- Augment therapeutic treatment for hypertension

- Relieve symptoms of migraine headaches

- Relieve asthma symptoms

- Assist in recovery from addiction by reducing withdrawal symptoms and promoting a clean and sober lifestyle

- Enhance sports performance

- Boost creativity

- Aid in conflict resolution

- Help resolve relationship problems

- Improve time management and efficiency

- Improve communication skills

- Foster positive habits and behaviors

Mental Imagery Steps

1. Assume a comfortable position and relax.

2. Adjust to receive the mental image created.

3. Select a pleasant visual theme for the image.

4. Allow your mind to enhance the image.

5. Utilize all senses to hear, see, touch, taste, and smell the image that has been brought to life in your mind.

6. Savor the image and calmly breathe.

MEDITATION

Meditation involves concentrating the mind to empty and cleanse it of stressful thoughts and ego-based worries. The focus of meditation is on internal rather than external control (Gawande et al., 2018). Meditation, a centuries-old technique that originated in Asia in the 6th century BCE, brings increased awareness and inner peace. It also lowers the heart rate and blood pressure, reduces oxygen consumption, and decreases muscle tension to improve physical and mental well-being (Balconi, Fronda, & Crivelli, 2018); improves skin integrity; and assists in brain processing (Benson & Klipper, 1992).

There are two types of meditation, although both involve concentrating to empty and cleanse the mind (Travis et al., 2018):

- **Exclusive or restrictive meditation.** This involves restricting the consciousness to focus on a single thought (Travis et al., 2018). Often this thought is a *mantra*—a one-syllable word such as "om" or "peace" that is repeated over and over to induce a tranquil meditative state. This clears other turbulent thoughts from the consciousness. One form of exclusive meditation is transcendental meditation.

- **Inclusive or opening-up meditation.** With this type of meditation, the mind is allowed to wander aimlessly, similar to free association. No topic or random spontaneous thought is off-limits. However, all thoughts must be observed objectively and without bias, judgment, or emotional directive (Balconi et al., 2018; Seaward, 2012). Inclusive meditation is also called access meditation, insightful meditation, or mindfulness meditation. Mindfulness meditation is described as a mental state characterized by full attention to internal and external perceptions of the present moment (Travis et al., 2018). Zen is a form of inclusive meditation.

Meditation Steps

1. Sit in the lotus position, with the legs crossed and folded, the wrists resting on the thighs, the palms open upward, and the thumb and index finger joined to capture the flow of the Earth's energy and direct it into the body. (See Figure 6.2.)

2. Begin repeating your mantra to induce higher levels of concentration.

3. Focus your vision on an object, such as a seashell, for 60 seconds.

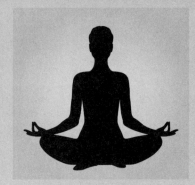

FIGURE 6.2 The lotus position.

4. Close your eyes and visualize the seashell to induce a calm and tranquil state.

5. Listen to repeated sounds, such as from a drum, a waterfall, or bells, to focus the mind.

6. Concentrate on the simple repetitive motion of your own breath until you can blot out the whole world and you are filled with peace.

7. Repeatedly rub the seashell or a smooth stone while holding it in your hand. Focus on the texture or smoothness of the object and exclude all other thoughts to transcend to a meditative state. This is called tactile repetition (Seaward, 2012; Zhao et al., 2018).

PROGRESSIVE MUSCULAR RELAXATION

Progressive muscular relaxation (PMR) involves tensing and relaxing muscle groups while also performing breathing exercises. PMR operates under the precept that the gradual contraction and relaxation of specific muscle groups promotes physical relaxation (Novais, Batista, Grazziano, & Amorim, 2016).

☑ **NOTE** PMR was developed during the early 20th century by Edmund Jacobson as a way to reduce or prevent tension-related illnesses. It was one of the first relaxation techniques ever developed in the United States.

With PMR, you contract each muscle group in your body, one at a time, starting with the muscles in your face (forehead, eyes, and jaw), ending with the muscles in your feet, and everything in between (jaw, neck, shoulders, upper chest, hands and forearms, abdomen, lower back, buttocks, thighs, and calves). (When applicable, contract both sides of the muscle group at the same time—for example, both shoulders, both forearms, both hands, and so on.) At the same time, you perform breathing exercises, inhaling deeply as you contract the muscle and exhaling as you relax it. While the muscle is relaxed, you compare how it feels with how it felt when it was contracted (Novais et al., 2016; Seaward, 2012).

> **❓ TIP** When doing PMR, choose an environment with minimal distractions and a comfortable room temperature.

PMR is beneficial both psychologically and physiologically. It reduces the fight-or-flight response, lessens tension, and promotes calm for optimal well-being. The technique is particularly helpful for defusing anger. Indeed, PMR is considered to be one of the most beneficial interventions for de-escalating angry individuals.

PMR Steps

1. Assume a comfortable sitting or lying-down position.

2. Inhale deeply and contract the muscles in your forehead and around your eyes for 5 to 10 seconds.

3. Exhale and relax for 45 seconds. Compare how the muscles feel now to how they felt when they were contracted.

4. Repeat steps 2 and 3, but this time, contract the muscles 50%.

5. Repeat step 4, but this time, contract the muscles 5%.

6. Repeat steps 2–5 with your jaw and then your neck.

7. Repeat steps 2–5 with your shoulders, contracting both at the same time.

8. Repeat steps 2–5 with your upper chest.

9. Repeat steps 2–5 with your hands, contracting both at the same time.

10. Repeat steps 2–5 with your forearms, contracting both at the same time.

11. Repeat steps 2–5 with your abdominals and then your lower back.

12. Repeat steps 2–5 with your buttocks, contracting both at the same time.

13. Repeat steps 2–5 with your thighs, contracting both at the same time.

14. Repeat steps 2–5 with your calves, contracting both at the same time.

15. Repeat steps 2–5 with your feet, contracting both at the same time.

REFERENCES

American Psychological Association. (2012). *Stress by generation.* Retrieved from https://www.apa.org/news/press/releases/stress/2012/generations

Anagnostouli, M., Babili, I., Chrousos, G., Artemiadis, A., & Darviri, C. (2018). A novel cognitive-behavioral stress management method for multiple sclerosis. A brief report of an observational study. *Neurological Research, 41*(3), 223–226. doi: 10.1080/01616412.2018.1548745

Arnetz, J. E., Hamblin,L., Essenmacher, L., Upfal, M. J., Ager, J., & Luborsky, M. (2015). Understanding patient-to-worker violence in hospitals: A qualitative analysis of documented incident reports. *Journal of Advanced Nursing, 71*(2), 338–348. doi: 10.1111/jan.12494

Balconi, M., Fronda, G., & Crivelli, D. (2018). Effects of technology-mediated mindfulness practice on stress: Psychophysiological and self-report measures. *Stress, 1–10.* doi: 10.1080/10253890.2018.1531845

Beizaee, Y., Rejeh, N., Heravi-Karimooi, M., Tadrisi, S. D., Griffiths, P., & Vaismoradi, M. (2018). The effect of guided imagery on anxiety, depression, and vital signs in patients on hemodialysis. *Complementary Therapies in Clinical Practice, 33,* 184–190. doi: 10.1016/j.ctcp.2018.10.008

Benson, H., & Klipper, Z. (1992). *The relaxation response.* Garden City, NY: Wings Books.

Bronk, K. L. (2019, January 29). Joint Commission issues new Quick Safety advisory on de-escalating aggression/agitation in health care settings. *The Joint Commission.* Retrieved from https://www.jointcommission.org/joint_commission_issues_new_quick_safety_advisory_on_de-escalating_aggressionagitation_in_health_care_settings/

Buhmann, C., Jungnickel, D., & Lehmann, E. (2018). Stress management training (SMT) improves coping of tremor-boosting psychosocial stressors and depression in patients with Parkinson's disease: A controlled prospective study. *Parkinson's Disease.* https://doi.org/10.1155/2018/4240178

Cohen, B. E., Edmondson, D., & Kronish, I. M. (2015). State of the art review: Depression, stress, anxiety, and cardiovascular disease. *American Journal of Hypertension, 28*(11), 1,295–1,302. doi: 10.1093/ajh/hpv047

Edwards, M. K., & Loprinzi, P. D. (2018). Experimental effects of brief, single bouts of walking and meditation on mood profile in young adults. *Health Promotion Perspectives, 8*(3), 171–178.

Edwards, M. K., Rhodes, R. E., Mann, J. R., & Loprinzi, P. D. (2018). Effects of acute aerobic exercise or meditation on emotional regulation. *Physiology & Behavior, 186,* 16–24. doi: 10.1016/j.physbeh.2017.12.037

Esler, M. (2017). Mental stress and human cardiovascular disease. *Neuroscience and Biobehavioral Reviews, 74*(Pt B), 269–276. doi: 10.1016/j.neubiorev.2016.10.011

Fiandaca, M. S., Mapstone, M., Connors, E., Jacobson, M., Monuki, E., Malik, S., ... Federoff, H. J. (2017). Systems healthcare: A holistic paradigm for tomorrow. *BMC Systems Biology, 11*, 142. doi: 10.1186/s12918-017-0521-2

Gawande, R., To, M. N., Pine, E., Griswold, T., Creedon, T. B., Brunel, A., ... Schuman-Olivier, Z. (2018). Mindfulness training enhances self-regulation and facilitates health behavior change for primary care patients: A randomized controlled trial. *Journal of General Internal Medicine, 34*(2), 293–302. doi: 10.1007/s11606-018-4739-5

Gillespie, G. L., Gates, D. M., Miller, M., & Howard, P. K. (2010). Workplace violence in healthcare settings: Risk factors and protective strategies. *Rehabilitation Nursing, 35*(5), 177–184.

Grossert, A., Urech, C., Alder, J., Gaab, J., Berger, T., & Hess, V. (2016). Web-based stress management for newly diagnosed cancer patients (STREAM-1): A randomized, wait-list controlled intervention study. *BMC Cancer, 16*(1), 838.

International Council of Nurses. (2007). *Guidelines on coping with violence in the workplace.* Retrieved from https://static1.squarespace.com/static/579770cd197aea84455d6908/t/57d86302d1758e16f4e0f072/1473798914990/guideline_violence.pdf

The Joint Commission. (2018). *Sentinel event alert 59: Physical and verbal violence against health care workers.* Retrieved from https://www.jointcommission.org/sea_issue_59/

Jung, C. G. (1964). *Man and his symbols.* New York, NY: Anchor Press.

Keane, P. (2006). How to de-escalate potentially aggressive interactions with patients. *Synergy,* 8–10.

Ketchesin, K. D., Stinnett, G. S., & Seasholtz, A. F. (2017). Corticotropin-releasing hormone-binding protein and stress: From invertebrates to humans. *Stress, 20*(5), 449–464. doi: 10.1080/10253890.2017.1322575

Li, A. W., & Goldsmith, C. A. (2012). The effects of yoga on anxiety and stress. *Alternative Medicine Review, 17*(1), 21–35.

Lown, B. A., & Setnik, G. S. (2018). Utilizing compassion and collaboration to reduce violence in healthcare settings. *Israel Journal of Health Policy, 7,* 39. doi: 10.1186/s13584-018-0234-z

Novais, P. G. N., Batista, K. D., Grazziano, E. D., & Amorim, M. H. C. (2016). The effects of progressive muscular relaxation as a nursing procedure used for those who suffer from stress due to multiple sclerosis. *Revista Latino-Americana de Enfermagen, 24,* e2,789. doi: 10.1590/ doi: 10.1590/1518-8345.1257.27891518-8345.1257.2789

Power, G. A. (2010). *Dementia beyond drugs: Changing the culture of care,* Baltimore, MD: Health Professions Press.

Sahranavard, V. S., Esmaeili, A., Dastjerdi, R., & Salehiniya, H. (2018). The effectiveness of stress-management-based cognitive-behavioral treatments on anxiety sensitivity, positive and negative affect and hope. *BioMedicine, 8*(4), 23. doi: 10.1051/bmdcn/2018080423

Seaward, B. L. (2012). *Managing stress: Principles and strategies for health and well-being* (7th ed.). Burlington, VT: Jones & Bartlett Learning.

Smith, C., Hancock, H., Blake-Mortimer, J., & Eckert, K. (2007). A randomized comparative trial of yoga and relaxation to reduce stress and anxiety. *Complementary Therapies in Medicine, 15*(2), 77–83.

Stefanaki, C., Bacopoulou, F., Livadas, S., Kandaraki, A., Karachalios, A., Chrousos, G. P., & Diamanti-Kandarakis, E. (2015). Impact of a mindfulness stress management program on stress, anxiety, depression and quality of life in women with polycystic ovary syndrome: A randomized controlled trial. *Stress, 18*(1), 57–66. doi: 10.3109/10253890.2014.974030

Travis, F., Valosek, L., Konrad, A., Link, J., Salerno, J., Scheller, R., & Nidich, S. (2018). Effect of meditation on psychological distress and brain functioning: A randomized controlled study. *Brain and Cognition, 125*, 100–105. doi: 10.1016/j.bandc.2018.03.011

Vinstrup, J., Jakobsen, M. D., Calatayud, J., Jay, K., & Andersen, L. L. (2018). Association of stress and musculoskeletal pain with poor sleep: Cross-sectional study among 3,600 hospital workers. *Frontiers in Neurology, 9*, 968. doi: 10.3389/fneur.2018.00968

Yong, M. S., Lee, Y. S., & Lee, H. Y. (2018). Effects of breathing exercises on resting metabolic rate and maximal oxygen uptake. *Journal of Physical Therapy Science, 30*(9), 1,173–1,175.

Yu, N., Chan, J. S. M., Ji, X., Wan, A. H. Y., Ng, S. M., Yuen, L. P., … Chan, C. H. Y. (2019). Stress and psychosomatic symptoms in Chinese adults with sleep complaints: Mediation effect of self-compassion. *Psychology, Health & Medicine, 24*(2), 241–252. doi: 10.1080/13548506.2018.1546014

Zhao, J., Li, X., Xiao, H., Cui, N., Sun, L., & Xu, Y. (2018). Mindfulness and burnout among bedside registered nurses: A cross-sectional study. *Nursing Health Sciences, 21*(1), 126–131. doi: 10.1111/nhs.12582

7

CONFLICT RESOLUTION

"Pursuing peace means rising above one's own wants, needs, and emotions."
–Benazir Bhutto

OBJECTIVES

- Identify two primary types of conflict

- Examine conflict-resolution styles

- Identify the elements of conflict resolution

- Explain the benefits of conflict resolution

In today's high-stress world, conflict is unavoidable. If we are living and breathing, we *will* encounter conflict. Busy healthcare environments are rife with conflict. Conflicts encountered in healthcare environments may include patient-nurse, patient-patient, patient–family member, nurse-nurse, nurse–interdisciplinary staff, and others. Katz and Lawyer (1993) define *conflict* as a situation or state involving two or more parties in which differences exist that are viewed by both or all parties as negative. Often, conflict is the spark that ignites agitation, aggression, or violence.

Healthcare environments abound with opportunities for conflict. Indeed, conflict in healthcare environments is inevitable. Healthcare environments contain multiple healthcare staff, patients, and visitors, all experiencing countless interactions in which conflict can arise at any time. *Conflict resolution* is a communication process used to settle conflict. It involves the use of negotiation to reach a solution that is agreeable to all parties.

Educating healthcare professionals in conflict resolution can prevent negative impacts due to conflict (Kfouri & Lee, 2019). Conflict-resolution skills are essential for nurses and other healthcare providers to reduce or prevent inpatient aggression and violence. Although conflict may exist in every aspect of our day-to-day lives—including in a healthcare environment—it's possible to mediate and settle conflict through the conflict-resolution process (Boca, Garro, Giammusso, & Abbate, 2018; Marshall & Robson, 2005).

> ☑ **NOTE** Not all conflict is bad. When managed effectively, conflict can lead to positive outcomes for nurses, patients, and colleagues and drive personal, professional, and organizational growth (Boyd, 2008). Conflict also gives nurses an opportunity to demonstrate respect for their patients, colleagues, and profession as a whole as they navigate the conflict-resolution process.

BENEFITS OF CONFLICT RESOLUTION

When effectively implemented, the conflict-resolution process offers substantial benefits. Not only does it resolve conflict, it also fosters a safe workplace, prevents violence, and improves patient and nurse morale. Eliminating the causes of discord also results in better nurse and group cohesion for improved quality of patient care and patient care outcomes (Baggs, Ryan, Phelps, Richeson, &

Johnson, 1992), allows for increased understanding between patients and nurses, and enhances therapeutic rapport. Finally, removing the tension and stress that naturally arise due to conflicts in the healthcare environment decreases staff turnover and improves patient and employee satisfaction.

TYPES OF CONFLICT

There are two main types of conflict (Katz & Lawyer, 1993):

- **Overt conflict.** This is conflict that is out in the open. With overt conflict, the conflicting parties tend to perceive their differences as irreconcilable and all possible outcomes as incompatible. These inalienable differences often fester into anger and hostility and may even result in violence (Occupational Safety and Health Administration, 2016).

- **Covert conflict.** This is conflict that goes unacknowledged or even occurs outside the psychological awareness of those involved (Katz & Lawyer, 1993). It manifests in powerful undercurrents of volatile emotions. Although covert conflict hides in the shadows, it causes disagreements and difficult-to-resolve issues. Until these conflicts are brought out into the open, they will remain as divisive instruments, potentiating agitation, aggression, and violence as a harsh result of unmet needs.

CONFLICT-RESOLUTION STYLES

There are many conflict-resolution styles, each with its own focus and method of resolution. As shown in Figure 7.1, conflict-resolution styles fall on a spectrum with regard to the levels of assertiveness and cooperation. The styles are as follows:

- **Avoiding.** This style is the lowest on the scale in both assertiveness and cooperation. With this style, all parties ignore the conflict (Thomas & Kilmann, 2008). Nurses frequently use this approach (Losa Iglesias & Becerro de Bengoa Vallejo, 2012). Unfortunately, it is a lose-lose strategy, and therefore the worst conflict-resolution style. Avoiding the conflict not only demonstrates an unwillingness to cooperate and communicate, it typically results in the conflict growing until it snowballs out of control.

CONFLICT RESOLUTION STYLES

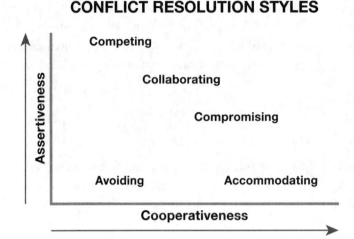

FIGURE 7.1 Conflict-resolution styles. (Adapted from Thomas & Kilmann, 2008.)

- **Competing.** This style is highest on the scale of assertiveness and lowest in cooperation. With this style, one party forces its will on the other party. This is a win-lose strategy. Although this conflict-resolution style may temporarily settle the conflict, it will likely result in resentments that could cause more conflicts down the line (Thomas & Kilmann, 2008). The only time this style is truly beneficial is when the conflict needs to be resolved immediately and there is no time to confer with the other parties in the conflict.

- **Collaborating.** This style is high in both assertiveness and cooperation. With this style, all parties involved in the conflict get together to work through the issue until they reach a solution that is agreeable to all. This conflict-resolution style relies on a clear positive vision and involves the use of problem-solving techniques to ensure that the interests of all parties are met (Losa Iglesias & Becerro de Bengoa Vallejo, 2012; Thomas & Kilmann, 2008). Collaborating is a win-win strategy and is therefore the best conflict-resolution style.

- **Compromising.** This style is in the middle of the scale in terms of both assertiveness and cooperation. With this style, each party gives a little bit of ground until they reach a median solution that satisfies everyone at least partially (Thomas & Kilmann, 2008). A mini-win–mini-win strategy is one of the better conflict-resolution styles.

■ **Accommodating.** With this style, one party yields completely to the other party to protect the relationships involved (Thomas & Kilmann, 2008). This is a lose-win strategy. This style is low on the spectrum with regard to assertiveness but high on the spectrum in terms of cooperation. This style is generally not beneficial unless preserving the relationship with the other party is more important that "winning" the conflict (hence its frequent use in marriages), as it often results in lingering resentment on the losing side.

> ✓ **NOTE** The desired outcome of any conflict-resolution effort is a win-win.

ELEMENTS OF CONFLICT RESOLUTION

There are several key elements to the conflict-resolution process. These elements can be arranged into an easy-to-remember acronym: CONFLICT. The elements that compose a holistic conflict-resolution model are as follows:

■ **Calmness.** Effective conflict resolution involves calmly addressing the underlying problem. There are several ways to achieve this. One is to choose a calm, quiet, and private setting to discuss the issue at hand—one that is away from other patients (but still within sight of other staff for safety reasons). Another is to take time to calm yourself and organize your thoughts before engaging the individuals in conflict (Liu, Wang, Quan, & Li, 2015). Finally, avoid taking a threatening stance, such as by standing over the patient, pointing your finger, placing your hands on your hips, or crossing your arms (McKibben, 2017; Rahim & Magner, 1995). The idea is to demonstrate an open attitude to address the conflict and to foster a calm atmosphere based in mutual respect.

■ **Objective professional approach:** While working through the conflict, take an objective and professional approach. To achieve this, you need to get a handle on how you react to conflict and take steps to temper these reactions if needed. Also, keep in mind that people often exchange cruel words in the heat of an argument but don't *really* mean them—meaning you need not take them to heart. At the same time, avoid making remarks to patients that are blaming, are threatening, or project guilt (Maurer, 1991), and avoid using your authority as a healthcare professional to impose your beliefs on others.

■ **Negotiate solutions.** Not all conflicts can be resolved, but negotiating with the other parties greatly increases your chances of success. Begin by working together to brainstorm all possible solutions, writing them down as you go. Then go back through the list and rate each solution from best to worst (Fletcher, 2019; Maurer, 1991). Be willing to compromise and meet the other party in the middle (Eisemann, Wagner, & Reece, 2018), splitting the difference until you reach a solution.

■ **Focus on the problem at hand.** During the conflict-resolution process, don't allow yourself to become distracted. Focus on the problem underlying the conflict—*not* on unrelated issues (Liu, Wang, Quan, & Li, 2015).

■ **Listen.** Every conflict has at least two sides. As you engage in the conflict-resolution process, it's imperative that you listen to all of them. Listen closely to what both parties say, and demonstrate that you understand the perspectives of all involved (Falkenhagen, 2006). Don't hurry either party. Give people time to voice their side of the conflict. Ask questions to clear up any confusing communications. Finally, acknowledge that all parties have the right to disagree.

■ **Initiate evaluation.** After the conflict-resolution process is complete, initiate a follow-up evaluation to assess its effectiveness. This enables you to determine whether the intervention worked and to monitor any progress made (Gundrosen, Thomassen, Wisborg, & Aadahl, 2018). It also demonstrates your commitment to resolving the conflict. If you determine that the intervention failed, consider contacting an independent third party to assist with mediation efforts. Sometimes, an outside person's viewpoint can be the catalyst for a successful solution.

■ **Communicate.** Conflict resolution requires clear communication (College of Nurses of Ontario, 2009). When communicating about a conflict, use techniques such as restating and clarifying to ensure proper understanding (Marshall & Robson, 2005). When all parties agree on a solution to the conflict, respectfully communicate the proposed change to affirm your commitment. For example, say, "In the future, I will show you the medication wrapper before I place the pills in your medication cup." Finally, document the solution and communicate it to the team to ensure its implementation (McKibben, 2017).

■ **Take a close look.** Examine the situation to determine whether additional or alternative interventions are required to resolve the conflict. If so, consider whether an impartial mediator or arbitrator might be able to facilitate a resolution. Never shy away from engaging a third party who might be able to break through and resolve the dispute. Research indicates that the level of hostility decreases most when mediation is accompanied by perspective-taking (Boca et al., 2018). If the conflict has already been successfully resolved, consider how to apply what you've learned during the conflict-resolution process to prevent similar conflicts from arising in the future.

> ✓ **NOTE** Resolving conflicts takes time, practice, and patience.

RULES FOR OPEN COMMUNICATION

Open communication is key to resolving any conflict. Here are a few rules for open communication to keep in mind:

■ Give each party a chance to tell their side of the story.

■ Allow all parties to express their anger.

■ Encourage the use of "I" statements. For example, the statement "I believe Anthony is taunting me" is less accusatory than "Anthony is taunting me."

■ Look for areas of agreement (Caplan, 1970) or views that all parties have in common.

■ Stay on topic. When one party is speaking, do not change the subject (Hosley & Molle-Matthews, 2006).

■ To encourage understanding among all parties, rephrase and repeat back what each person says.

■ If one person's position is unclear, ask questions to clarify it.

> ✓ **NOTE** Cooperation and collaboration are key to conflict resolution.

REFERENCES

Baggs, J. G, Ryan, S. A., Phelps, C. E., Richeson, J. F., & Johnson, J. E. (1992). The association between interdisciplinary collaboration and patient outcomes in a medical intensive care unit. *Heart and Lung: The Journal of Critical Care, 21*(1), 18–24.

Boca, S., Garro, M., Giammusso, I., & Abbate, C. S. (2018). The effect of perspective taking on the mediation process. *Psychology Research and Behavioral Management, 11,* 411–416. doi: 10.2147/PRBM.S168956

Boyd, M. A. (2008). *Psychiatric nursing: Contemporary practice* (4th ed.). Philadelphia, PA: Lippincott, Williams & Wilkins.

Caplan, G. (1970). *The theory and practice of mental health consultation.* New York, NY: Basic Books, Inc.

College of Nurses of Ontario. (2009). *Conflict prevention and management.* Toronto, ON: College of Nurses of Ontario.

Eisemann, B. S., Wagner, R. D., & Reecc, E. M. (2018). Practical negotiation for medical professionals. *Seminars in Plastic Surgery, 32*(4), 166–171.

Falkenhagen, K. (2006). *Conflict resolution skills in nursing.* Homestead Schools Inc.: Torrance, CA.

Fletcher, J. R. (2019). Negotiating tensions between methodology and procedural ethics. *Journal of Gerontological Social Work, 6,* 1–8.

Gundrosen, S., Thomassen, G., Wisborg, T., & Aadahl, P. (2018). Team talk team decision processes: A qualitative discourse analytical approach to 10 real-life medical emergency team encounters. *British Medical Journal, 8*(11). https://bmjopen.bmj.com/content/8/11/e023749

Hosley, J., & Molle-Matthews, E. (2006). *A practical guide to therapeutic communication for healthcare professionals.* St. Louis, MO: Saunders.

Katz, N. H., & Lawyer, J. W. (1993). *Conflict resolution: Building bridges.* Thousand Oaks, CA: Corwin Press Inc.

Kfouri, J., & Lee, P. E. (2019). Conflict among colleagues: Health care providers feel undertrained and unprepared to manage inevitable workplace conflict. *Journal of Obstetrics and Gynaecology Canada, 41*(1), 15–20. doi: 10.1016/j.jogc.2018.03.132

Liu, Y., Wang, Z., Quan, S., & Li, M. (2015). The effect of positive affect on conflict resolution: Modulated by approach-motivational intensity. *Cognition & Emotion, 31*(1), 69–82.

Losa Iglesias, M. E., & Becerro de Bengoa Vallejo, R. (2012). Conflict resolution styles in the nursing profession. *Contemporary Nurse, 43*(1), 73–80. doi: 10.5172/conu.2012.43.1.73

Marshall, P., & Robson, R. (2005). Preventing and managing conflict: Vital pieces in the patient safety puzzle. *Healthcare Quarterly, 8,* 39–44.

Maurer, R. E. (1991). *Managing conflict: Tactics for school administrators.* Boston, MA: Allyn and Bacon.

McKibben, L. (2017). Conflict management: Importance and implications. *British Journal of Nursing, 26*(2), 100–103. doi: 10.12968/bjon.2017.26.2.100

Occupational Safety and Health Administration. (2016). Guidelines for preventing workplace violence for health care & social service workers. *OSHA.* Retrieved from http://www.osha.gov/Publications/osha3148.pdf

Rahim, M. A., & Magner, N. R. (1995). Confirmatory factor analysis of the styles of handling interpersonal conflict: First-order factor model and its invariance across groups. *Journal of Applied Psychology, 80*(1), 122–132.

Thomas, K. W., & Kilmann, R. H. (2008). Thomas-Kilmann conflict mode instrument. *The Myers-Briggs Company*. Retrieved from https://shop.themyersbriggs.com/en/tkiitems.aspx?ic=4813&krs=kmyh4515ckvtnfmg2r5f43pa

8

CRISIS INTERVENTION

"Peace is a gift to each other."
–Elie Wiesel

OBJECTIVES

- Note the stages of crisis development

- Identify common behaviors in a crisis state

- Explain types of crises

- Discuss three phases of crisis intervention

- Identify key communication skills and practices for crisis intervention

Stress is rampant in our modern world. All too often, this stress escalates to a crisis. A *crisis* is a debilitating imbalance in one's internal equilibrium caused by a sudden stressor or threat to the self (Boyd, 2008). When people experience an overwhelmingly stressful life event with which they are unable to cope, a crisis is often the result (Flannery & Everly, 2000).

People in crisis can be found everywhere, including in healthcare facilities (Allen, Currier, Hughes, Reyes-Harde, & Docherty, 2001). Indeed, nurses frequently encounter people in crisis—whether they are patients, family members, or even other staff. Therefore, some of the most useful skills a nurse can have are crisis-intervention skills. *Crisis-intervention skills* are therapeutic skills used to intervene successfully and safely with individuals in crisis (Townsend, 2015).

> ☑ **NOTE** Nurses in regular healthcare facilities encounter individuals in crisis more often than nurses in mental health facilities. This is because many people in regular healthcare facilities are being treated for serious injuries or catastrophic illnesses—both common causes of crisis.

STAGES OF CRISIS DEVELOPMENT

Caplan (1970) describes crises as developing in four distinct stages, beginning with a stressor and ending in a panic state. The stages are as follows:

1. The patient is exposed to an overpowering precipitating stressor. In response, the patient attempts to remove the stressor for relief of discomfort.

2. The patient is unable to remove the stressor and unable to cope with the discomfort. Anxiety begins to build.

3. The patient activates all available internal and external resources at a maximum level to remove the stressor.

4. The patient is unable to remove the stressor, and anxiety builds to a panic level. Cognitive functioning is impaired, emotions become labile (mood swings), and behavior caused by psychotic thinking may emerge.

Crisis states are generally not chronic or long-term in nature. Indeed, the human body cannot maintain a crisis state indefinitely. Most crises are self-limiting, lasting no longer than four to six weeks.

COMMON CRISIS STATE BEHAVIORS

When people are in a crisis state, they may display certain specific characteristic behaviors. Knowing what these characteristic behaviors are can help nurses identify when someone is in a crisis state. These characteristic behaviors include the following:

- The person appears agitated, disturbed, tense, or anxious, with increasing levels of emotional distress (perhaps indicated by uncontrollable crying).

- The person exhibits a decline in overall cognitive function, losing the ability to concentrate or think clearly, becoming overwhelmed by emotional stress.

- The person becomes confused or forgetful or exhibits disorganized thinking (Varcarolis, 2011).

- The person experiences poor impulse control.

- The person becomes socially withdrawn.

- The person exhibits increased psychomotor activity—for example, running around aimlessly.

- The person experiences perceptual changes and intense feelings (Caplan, 1970).

- The person experiences flashbacks, intrusive thoughts, or nightmares.

In advanced crisis states, people may suffer hallucinations, depending on the severity and intensity of the stressor. People in crisis may also experience suicidal or homicidal ideations. Healthcare professionals should complete a risk assessment to determine whether these conditions exist and provide safety interventions as needed (Boyd, 2008). (See Chapter 10, "Performing a Mental Status Assessment," for details.)

> ✅ **NOTE** Often, people in a crisis state are isolated from usual sources of support, such as family or friends. In fact, this may predispose the person to enter into a crisis state.

TYPES OF CRISES

Townsend (2015) has identified six types of crises. Each type can inflict significant emotional upheaval in an individual's life. The six types of crises are as follows:

- **Dispositional crisis.** A dispositional crisis occurs when a specific external event upsets equilibrium (Zanello, Berthoud, & Bacchetta, 2017)—for example, breaking up with one's significant other or the loss of a loved one. This type of crisis can be emotionally devastating for those lacking emotional support and coping skills.

- **Anticipated life crisis.** An anticipated life crisis results from life challenges with both present and future implications. This type of crisis is often caused by a change in lifestyle—for example, getting married. Often, when one marries, one focuses on future responsibilities, such as having children. This can precipitate a crisis.

- **Traumatic stress.** This type of crisis may occur in the aftermath of a particularly devastating sudden, accidental, or unexpected traumatic event. An example of such an event might be an automobile accident that results in the death of one or more family members, bringing overwhelming grief, turmoil, and suffering (Lating & Bono, 2008; Li & Xu, 2012).

- **Maturational/developmental.** A maturational/developmental crisis occurs when an individual transitions from one age group to another, such as an adolescent transitioning into young adulthood or a young adult transitioning to older adulthood. The source of the crisis is the stress that comes with adopting the roles and responsibilities associated with the new life phase. A maturational/developmental crisis can occur at any transition point in aging.

- **Crisis reflecting psychopathology.** A crisis reflecting psychopathology is one caused by the presence of a preexisting severe mental disorder such as bipolar disorder, an anxiety disorder, borderline personality disorder, or schizophrenia (Murphy, Irving, Adams, & Driver, 2012). For example, some symptoms of severe mental illness, such as visual and auditory hallucinations in schizophrenia, can trigger a crisis.

> ☑ **NOTE** Individuals who suffer from mental illness are at higher risk of experiencing a crisis. This is because they may be more susceptible to life stressors that precipitate crisis. They may also lack the adaptive coping responses needed to handle a crisis.

- **Psychiatric emergency.** A psychiatric emergency is a situation in which an individual's general functioning is severely impaired. In this type of crisis, the individual is rendered incompetent or unable to resume normal intellectual functioning. Psychiatric emergencies may result from acute suicidal ideation, drug overdose, alcohol intoxication, hallucinogenic use, active psychosis, or an acute delusional state (Regier et al., 1990). Psychiatric emergencies are frequently encountered in emergency departments as well as in mental health facilities.

THREE PHASES OF CRISIS INTERVENTION

The primary goal of any crisis intervention is to provide relief to the person in crisis to restore to a pre-crisis level of functioning or higher. Ideally, it might even initiate a new and healthier way of coping—one that is useful beyond the present crisis.

Caplan (1970) identified three phases of crisis intervention. These phases are as follows:

1. Develop an alliance

2. Gather information

3. Problem-solve

Developing an alliance is about building trust and rapport. Here are some ways to achieve this:

- Introduce yourself. State your name, role, and purpose for speaking with the patient.

- Ask the patient how to be addressed.

- Ensure the patient's physical and emotional safety.

- Ensure the patient's comfort—for example, by offering a warm blanket or a snack or beverage.

- Provide a private and relaxing environment to help keep the patient calm and to enable the patient to gather thoughts.

- Speak quietly to the patient in a soothing manner.

- Begin where the patient wants to begin.

- Help the patient verbalize emotions about, reactions to, and perceptions of the event.

- Acknowledge the patient's feelings of helplessness.

- Don't leave the patient alone.

As you gather information, you'll want to find out as much as you can about the precipitating event. You'll also want to get a sense of the patient's medical history and personal circumstances. Here are some techniques to get the patient talking about the precipitating event:

- Ask open-ended questions to ascertain what triggered the crisis, such as "What happened?" "What is going on?" or "What is upsetting you?"

- Ask clarifying questions to pinpoint the nature of the crisis.

- Ask the patient to identify the most pressing problems, one at a time, until all have been vocalized (Caplan, 1970; Kneisl & Trigoboff, 2009).

- Review what you understand to be the primary and most pressing problem.

> ☑ **NOTE** Chapter 5, "Therapeutic Communication for De-Escalation," has more information about developing rapport and gathering information.

As for the patient's medical history and personal circumstances, you'll want to find out about the following:

- Current medications (some medications can cause paradoxical effects such as depression or agitation)

- Any history of medical, mental health, or substance abuse problems

- Any history or risk of harming behaviors

- The patient's cognitive status

- Past and present stressors

- Cultural factors that could affect the patient's circumstances

- Sources of emotional support such as a family member or trusted pastor

Problem-solving is about helping the person work through the crisis. Here are a few best practices:

- Ask the patient about having experienced a similar situation or crisis in the past and how it was handled then (Kercher, 1991).

- Ask the patient what stress-reduction techniques work best.

- Identify coping skills that might work for this situation to help the patient calm down (Calvert & Palmer, 2003).

- Ask questions to identify possible resolutions to the crisis.

- Help the patient brainstorm healthy alternatives to restore homeostasis.

- Don't give advice. Instead, provide information to motivate the person to make positive decisions. This helps build the person's self-esteem and self-respect.

- Set realistic goals (as identified by the individual).

- Pinpoint patient strengths (such as support from family and friends or spiritual support).

> **? TIP** As you speak to the patient, encourage slow, deep breaths. This can help reduce hyperventilation and panic responses.

THE IMPORTANCE OF COMMUNICATION DURING A CRISIS

It is important to have effective communication skills with patients in crisis (van Oenen et al., 2013). After all, it's communication skills that will enable you to develop an alliance, gather information, and help the patient problem-solve. The following communication skills are particularly important when faced with a person in crisis. (Chapter 5 describes many of these skills in more detail.)

- Establish a rapport.

- Show empathy.

- Show respect.

- Be available.

- Take clues from the patient's body language.

- Encourage verbalization.

- Use positive reinforcement.

Take a Team Approach

Use a team approach in crisis intervention. Engage the entire healthcare team, counselors, and a therapist (if available) to assist the person in crisis.

A social worker is another excellent resource for patients in crisis. Social workers are available on both medical and mental health units to assist patients. A social worker can greatly help patients experiencing psychosocial stressors. For example, social workers can help patients locate community resources such as housing, food, and parenting classes, which may substantially reduce patient stress and help to defuse a crisis.

Engaging ancillary disciplines such as social workers in a crisis is a vital intervention. This practice promotes homeostasis and de-escalates individuals with stressful psychosocial issues that trigger agitated behavior.

REFERENCES

Allen, M. H., Currier, G. W., Hughes, D. H., Reyes-Harde, M, & Docherty, J. P. (2001). The expert consensus guideline series: Treatment of behavioral emergencies. *Postgrad Medicine*, 1–88.

Boyd, M. A. (2008). *Psychiatric nursing: Contemporary practice* (4th ed.). Philadelphia, PA: Lippincott, Williams & Wilkins.

Calvert, P., & Palmer, C. (2003). Application of the cognitive therapy model to initial crisis assessment. *International Journal of Mental Health Nursing, 12*(1), 30–38.

Caplan, G. (1970). *The theory and practice of mental health consultation*. New York, NY: Basic Books, Inc.

Flannery, R. B., & Everly, G. S. (2000). Crisis intervention: A review. *International Journal of Emergency Mental Health, 2*(2), 119–125.

Kercher, E. E. (1991). Crisis intervention in the emergency department. *Emergency Medicine Clinics of North America, 9*(1), 219–232.

Kneisl, C. R., & Trigoboff, E. (2009). *Contemporary psychiatric-mental health nursing* (2nd ed.). Upper Saddle River, NJ: Prentice Hall.

Lating, J. M., & Bono, S. F. (2008). Crisis intervention and fostering resiliency. *International Journal of Emergency Mental Health, 10*(2), 87–93.

Li, Y., & Xu, Z. (2012). Psychological crisis intervention for the family members of patients in a vegetative state. *Clinics, 67*(4), 341–345. doi: 10.6061/clinics/2012(04)07

Murphy, S., Irving, C. B., Adams, C. E., & Driver, R. (2012). Crisis intervention for people with severe mental illnesses. *The Cochrane Database of Systematic Reviews.* doi: 10.1002/14651858.CD001087.pub4

Regier, D. A., Farmer, M. E., Rae, D. S., Locke, B. Z., Keith, S. J., Judd, L. L., & Goodwin, F. K. (1990). Comorbidity of mental disorders with alcohol and other drug abuse: Results from the Epidemiologic Catchment Area (ECA) study. *Journal of the American Medical Association, 264*(19), 2,511–2,518.

Townsend, M. C. (2015). *Psychiatric mental health nursing: Concepts of care in evidence-based practice* (8th ed.). Philadelphia, PA: F. A. Davis Company.

van Oenen, F. J., Schipper, S., Van, R., Schoevers, R., Visch, I., Peen, J., & Dekker, J. (2013). Efficacy of immediate patient feedback in emergency psychiatry: A randomized controlled trial in a crisis intervention & brief therapy team. *BMC Psychiatry, 13,* 331.

Varcarolis, E. M. (2011). *Manual of psychiatric nursing care planning: Assessment guides, diagnoses, psychopharmacology* (4th ed.). New York, NY: Elsevier Health Sciences.

Zanello, A., Berthoud, L., & Bacchetta, J. (2017). Emotional crisis in a naturalistic context: Characterizing outpatient profiles and treatment effectiveness. *BMC Psychiatry, 17,* 130. doi: 10.1186/s12888-017-1293-3

MANAGING MENTAL HEALTH EMERGENCIES

*"I do not want the peace which passeth understanding.
I want the understanding which bringeth peace."*

–Helen Keller

OBJECTIVES

- Identify common mental health emergencies

- Find out how to perform an emergency mental health assessment

- Learn about how to aid suicidal patients

- Examine how to help patients suffering from drug or alcohol dependency or abuse

- Discover how to assist violent patients

Mental health emergencies are considered to be any disturbance in thoughts, feelings, or actions for which immediate therapeutic intervention is needed. Common adult mental health emergencies include suicidal thoughts or behaviors; alcohol or substance abuse; aggressive behaviors; and mood, anxiety, and psychotic disorders (Kimble, 2008).

Mental health emergencies can occur in any healthcare setting, including clinics, hospitals, and emergency departments. Indeed, more than one-third of patients presenting to emergency departments are there due to mental health issues. Of these mental health emergencies (Stuart, 2009):

- An average of 20% are related to suicide and/or suicide attempts

- More than 10% are related to aggressive or violent behavior

- An estimated 1 million per year are related to drug or alcohol abuse or addictive disorders

Moreover, it is estimated that more than 40% of patients treated for mental health emergencies are hospitalized directly from the emergency department after triage (Stuart, 2009).

> ☑ **NOTE** Persons with mental health emergencies are distributed evenly according to sex.

Every year, the number of individuals presenting to emergency departments for psychiatric triage due to mental health issues increases. There are several reasons for this increase in mental health emergencies (which are more common in individuals with mental illness). One reason is the de-institutionalization of the chronically mentally ill. This has resulted in large numbers of severely chronically mentally ill patients living in the community rather than residing in mental hospitals as they did in the past. The de-institutionalized chronically mentally ill require frequent monitoring and follow-up care, which they often receive at local clinics, hospitals, and emergency departments.

Other reasons for the increase in the number of individuals seeking psychiatric triage include the following:

- **The general population is getting older.** This has brought about an increase in age-related illnesses such as dementia and toxic confusion.

▪ **There has been a surge in alcohol and substance abuse.** Recreational and addictive drug use is epidemic and often results in drug intoxication. Individuals suffering from this condition are often triaged and treated in clinics, hospitals, and emergency departments (Warren, 2009).

▪ **We live in a very stressful age.** Despite economic progress, people today seem to have more stressful lives than ever before. These stressed-out individuals frequently need psychiatric support as well as mental health counseling.

> ✅ **NOTE** Your goal when responding to any mental health emergency is to teach the patient effective coping strategies and to help the patient restore a sense of balance and self-control. When the patient returns back to regular life, you want functioning to be at a level equal to or even above pre-crisis levels.

COMMON MENTAL HEALTH EMERGENCIES

The three most common mental health emergencies that present in emergency departments are, in order:

▪ **Suicidal behavior.** Suicidal behavior (including ideation and attempts) stemming from depression is a frequent diagnosis in emergency departments (Nadler-Moodie, 2010; Stuart, 2009).

▪ **Drug and alcohol abuse.** The medical and psychological effects of substance abuse and addiction are a common reason for triage in emergency departments.

▪ **Domestic violence.** Often, this is related to psychosocial issues and substance abuse.

Other common mental health emergencies involve individuals with seriously impaired judgment that causes them to endanger themselves due to self-neglect or self-harming behaviors. Mental states that impair judgment may be caused by conditions such as delirium or dementia, by acute psychotic episodes, or by severe dissociative states (Kleespies, 1998; Varcarolis, 2011).

> ❓ **TIP** Often, patients who present in the emergency department for a mental health emergency are in a crisis state. For a list of crisis symptoms and how to respond, refer to Chapter 8, "Crisis Intervention."

PERFORMING AN EMERGENCY MENTAL HEALTH ASSESSMENT

To ensure patient safety, mental health emergencies are triaged immediately, and the patient is assessed to determine danger to self or others. Part of this assessment is the completion of lab tests and medical evaluations as ordered by the physician, including a urine screening for drugs and alcohol (Tintinalli, Kelen, & Stapczynski, 2000).

In addition, a comprehensive mental status assessment is completed in the emergency department by the clinician or provider upon patient admission. As noted in Chapter 10, "Performing a Mental Status Assessment," this assessment involves observing and documenting the following information about the patient:

- Physical appearance

- Alertness, orientation, attitude, affect, and mood

- Thought processes, thought content, attention, concentration, and memory

- Judgment, insight, and intellect

- The presence of hallucinations or delusions

- Speech and motor activity

This information can help clinicians determine whether the patient may be suffering from psychiatric symptoms and, if so, the severity of these symptoms.

> **? TIP** While interviewing the patient, be alert for both verbal and nonverbal forms of communication. Also identify any hidden social, environmental, and cultural factors that may be contributing to the immediate situation (Vergare, Binder, Cook, Galanter, & Lu, 2006).

The mental status assessment also involves risk assessments to determine whether the patient is a danger to himself (suicidal) or to others (violent or homicidal). (See Chapter 10 for specifics.)

A Review of Suicidal Indicators

The admitting provider should be aware of indicators of suicidal intent. As discussed in Chapter 10, these include the following:

- The patient describes feelings of overwhelming anxiety.

- The patient suddenly gives away all valuable property and treasured belongings.

- The patient's outlook suddenly seems "better." (This may indicate that the patient has made a decision and has the means for a successful suicide.)

- The patient begins telephoning or texting others to say goodbye or writes a suicide note.

When completing an emergency mental status assessment, it is vital to obtain pertinent information from all available sources of information. These sources of information could include the following (Kleespies, 1998):

- The patient

- The patient's family members

- Law enforcement (e.g., if the patient was a victim of a violent crime or of sexual assault)

A review of the patient's medical record can also provide important information to ascertain the patient's health status.

Following this is an in-depth assessment of the patient's history. The goals here are to:

- Identify potentially traumatizing events that could be contributing to the patient's distress. This could include an overwhelming life event such as the death of a close friend, spouse, or child.

- Assess whether the patient has a history of suicidal, violent, or homicidal ideation or behavior.

- Uncover any history of psychiatric disorders such as depression, personality disorders, bipolar disorder, schizophrenia, or anxiety disorders.

■ Reveal a history of any concurrent serious medical conditions or illnesses such as cancer, heart disease, uncontrolled diabetes, lupus, or multiple sclerosis.

If the emergency assessment reveals that the patient is stable, your next step is to determine whether you should discharge the patient to outpatient care or opt for partial hospitalization. If the assessment reveals that the patient is unstable, then crisis intervention and stabilization efforts are called for, followed by inpatient hospitalization for therapeutic treatment and recovery. You must also determine whether precautionary measures are needed to protect the patient or others from harm.

> ☑ **NOTE** Treatment planning and case management is implemented for both inpatient and outpatient care for optimal recovery outcomes.

Establishing Trust and Rapport

When interviewing a patient in the middle of a mental health emergency, you must employ an interview style that enables you to quickly establish trust and rapport. The most effective way to do this is to use active listening skills. This will help you grasp the crisis from the patient's perspective. It can also help you find out what is important to the patient in everyday life (Caplan, 1970). This information can help you forge a bond with the patient.

AIDING THE SUICIDAL PATIENT

As noted in Chapter 10, "Performing a Mental Status Assessment," and Chapter 11, "De-Escalation of Patients With Mental Disorders," if you determine that a patient is actively suicidal, you must admit that individual. You must also initiate constant one-on-one observation, in which one nurse constantly monitors one patient, to prevent self-harm, and implement the facility suicide prevention plan if one is available.

Methods of Suicide

Unfortunately, it's not just patients experiencing suicidal ideation who regularly present in emergency departments. Patients who have attempted suicide may also be admitted (assuming they are not dead on arrival). Sadly, many do not survive.

The most common methods of suicide are, in order:

1. **Firearm.** Firearms are used in 54% of successful suicides. In households with firearms, the rate for completed suicides is five times higher than in households without firearms.

2. **Suffocation.** Most often this is due to hanging and subsequent strangulation.

3. **Poisoning.** Medication overdose is the most common method of suicide by poisoning. In more than 50% of successful suicides by overdose, the prescription was either written or filled less than one week before the suicide (Centers for Disease Control and Prevention, 2011).

TEST YOURSELF

MENTAL HEALTH EMERGENCIES Mr. Allen is a 52-year-old man newly arrived at a community outpatient medical clinic. He is accompanied by his sister and brother. Mr. Allen has a history of bipolar disorder. Mr. Allen arrives alert, oriented, and well-dressed, but with a sad affect. Mr. Allen reveals that he is anxious, depressed, and despondent due to his recent divorce. He has a prior history of two previous serious suicide attempts, and family members say that Mr. Allen has again threatened suicide. Mr. Allen cries, "My wife has left me!" and "I don't want to live anymore!"

How would you handle this situation?

AIDING THE PATIENT SUFFERING FROM ALCOHOL OR SUBSTANCE ABUSE

After triage and assessment are completed on a patient suffering from alcohol or substance dependency or abuse, a determination must made as to next steps. There are three main options, depending on the severity of the patient's condition:

- A patient requiring detoxification can be transferred to an inpatient detoxification facility. Various private and public alcohol/substance abuse treatment facilities provide inpatient detoxification services. These usually involve between three and seven days of inpatient treatment (Henningfield, Santora, & Bickel, 2007).

- If the patient has a dual diagnosis of mental illness and alcohol dependency, the physician may offer a referral to a mental health facility that also provides detoxification services.

- If the patient is assessed as experiencing less severe alcohol abuse, such as occasional binge drinking, the physician may offer a referral to a support organization such as Alcoholics Anonymous (AA) or to an outpatient treatment facility such as a halfway house.

- If the patient is diagnosed with dependency on or abuse of other substances, the physician will advise attending one or more support groups such as Narcotics Anonymous (NA), Cocaine Anonymous (CA), or Marijuana Anonymous (MA).

> ✅ **NOTE** The disposition of the assessed patient plays a role in what happens here. That is to say, the patient must be agreeable to receiving treatment.

To determine the severity of a patient's dependency on alcohol use, caregivers frequently complete something called a CAGE questionnaire. The results of the CAGE questionnaire dictate detoxification protocols to prevent the advent of delirium tremens or seizures from alcohol withdrawal. CAGE stands for:

- Cut down

- Annoyed

- Guilty

- Eye-opener

Typical questions in a CAGE questionnaire are as follows (Townsend, 2015, p. 395):

- Have you ever felt the need to **cut down** on your drinking?

- Have you ever been **annoyed** by others criticizing your drinking?

- Have you ever felt **guilty** or upset about your drinking?

- Have you ever had to drink as an **eye-opener** first thing in the morning to steady your hands or your nerves or to get over a hangover?

The CAGE questionnaire is a vital assessment for emergency departments. Between 20% and 30% of emergency department admissions are related to alcohol, and 40% of individuals with mental health emergencies are hospitalized by way of the emergency department (Stuart, 2009).

Caring For Patients in Alcohol Withdrawal

When caring for patients in alcohol withdrawal, keep these points in mind:

- Administer prescribed detoxification medications to reduce severity of symptoms and prevent seizures.

- Implement fall and seizure precautions for safety.

- Promote good hygiene, rest, and sleep.

- Monitor food and fluid intake for adequate nutrition and hydration.

- Maintain a quiet, calm environment.

- Play soft music.

- Promote the use of relaxation techniques such as deep breathing and mental imagery for healing and recovery (Nadler-Moodie, 2010).

- Encourage supportive family members and others to stay at the bedside to provide emotional support.

- Reassure the patient of safety.

AIDING THE VIOLENT PATIENT

Violence is a common reason for a mental health evaluation and admission to a mental health facility. Between 10% and 40% of mental health admissions occur to address issues with aggression and violence (Singh, Fazel, Gueorguieva, & Buchanan, 2014; Swanson, 1994). It is important to understand, however, that violence toward others is *not* typical of the mentally ill. Indeed, violence even in its rawest form is considered aberrant behavior among this population. People who suffer from mental illness are far more likely to be victims of violence than to perpetrate it.

In any case, you de-escalate a violent patient using many of the same techniques as with any other aggressive patient. The most notable of these is verbal de-escalation. The idea is to encourage the patient to describe the precipitating events that caused the violent thoughts, plans, or behavior, keeping all pertinent points pertaining to effective therapeutic communication in mind. Diverting the patient's attention may also be effective.

With a violent patient, it's particularly important to stay calm, convey respect, set (and enforce) limits, establish trust, be truthful, keep your promises, and *never* issue threats. You'll also need to provide a private and quiet environment. This both helps the patient relax and ensures the safety of other patients. While you're at it, remove any objects from the patient's reach that could be used to inflict harm on the self or others.

If possible, it's best to use psychological de-escalation techniques with a violent patient. However, depending on the patient's behavioral control and ability to cooperate, you may need to assess the need for PRN (as needed) medications and initiate one-to-one observation with continuous monitoring and de-escalation. If all least-restrictive measures fail and the patient is a danger to self or others, restraints are an option only as a last resort and if applied and monitored as per facility policy for safety.

CASE STUDY

HANDLING A MENTAL HEALTH EMERGENCY

At 5:20 p.m., Lewis, a 34-year-old man with a history of schizophrenia, is brought into the ED by his parents for homicidal ideation. His parents tell the ER physician that Lewis recently broke up with his girlfriend and has been increasingly agitated ever since. Earlier in the day, Lewis reported hearing voices in his head and threatened to attack his parents and brother. His parents brought Lewis to the ED for a mental health evaluation.

When Lewis arrives at the ED triage area, he yells, "Who are you and what are you doing in my house?" and shoves two nurses to the floor. The ED physician commits Lewis involuntarily and contacts a mental health clinician to complete a mental status exam on the patient. While waiting for the mental health clinician to arrive, Lewis is placed in a private ED room with

a security guard sitting outside on a one-to-one basis for safety.

At 6:40 p.m. the mental health clinician arrives to complete the physician-ordered mental status assessment. The mental health clinician walks by the guard and enters the patient's room. Lewis has been pacing back and forth. When he sees the clinician, he leans forward, clenches both fists, and begins stomping toward her. The security guard and clinician recognize the body language of escalation and danger. The security guard activates the facility "buddy system." Four additional guards arrive as backup and stand behind him outside the patient's door. Meanwhile, the mental health clinician communicates with the patient. The clinician stands inside the patient's room one foot from the doorway, near the exit for safety.

The clinician knows the patient is agitated and that she must quickly show respect to establish therapeutic rapport and calm him down. The clinician makes eye contact with the patient and calmly states, "Sir, my name is Mary, and I am here to talk with you. Sir, what you feeling right now?"

Lewis straightens up, opens his hands, calms down, and stops pacing. He looks at the clinician and replies, "I feel like I am in another world, like I am in Oz."

"Sir, did you watch that movie when you were a child?" the clinician asks Lewis.

"Yes," says Lewis. "I loved *The Wizard of Oz*."

"Sir, did you watch *Casablanca*, too?" the clinician asks.

"Yes! Oh, Humphrey Bogart is my favorite actor." The patient's body language is now relaxed. He smiles and pulls up a stool to sit next to the clinician as they begin to calmly discuss old movies.

The additional security guards who had gathered as backup observe that the patient is calming down and disperse, the possible take-down having been averted. Only the required one-to-one security guard remains outside the door as required by hospital policy and physician order.

The clinician asks the patient the questions necessary to complete the mental status assessment. Interspersed between the mental status questions, the clinician and patient talk about their favorite old movies, developing a good therapeutic rapport. Finally, the mental status assessment is complete.

The clinician has developed such good rapport with the patient that she volunteers to accompany him to the psychiatric hospital to prevent the patient from becoming agitated during the transfer. After the patient is medically cleared by the ED physician, the clinician accompanies the patient to the transport van. The patient politely opens the van door for the clinician and helps her get seated.

After the patient arrives at the psychiatric facility and is safely situated behind the locked mental health unit doors, the clinician asks the patient what happened to change him from the person described to her in the report from the ED nurses. The clinician kindly says, "Sir, I heard that you physically assaulted two nurses in the ED. Sir, you seem like such a gentleman. What changed?"

The patient looks at her and says, "You were the only person in that place that talked to me like I was a human being." That was all the patient wanted: to be talked to like he was an ordinary person.

As healthcare professionals, we must remember to *not* feed into stigma associated with mental illness. When we as nurses see a psychiatric diagnosis on a patient's chart, we must remember the patient is a person for whom we have great hopes for recovery, and we must respect him. When you respect people, you teach them to respect themselves. When people can respect themselves, they can learn to respect others. Show respect in every interaction. With respect, you can help pull a patient out of a crisis and effectively de-escalate.

REFERENCES

Caplan, G. (1970). *The theory and practice of mental health consultation*. New York, NY: Basic Books, Inc.

Centers for Disease Control and Prevention. (2011). Violence prevention: Suicide. *Centers for Disease Control and Prevention*. Retrieved from https://www.cdc.gov/violenceprevention/suicide/index.html

Henningfield, J. E., Santora, P. B., & Bickel, W. K. (2007). *Addiction treatment: Science and policy for the twenty-first century*. Baltimore, MD: Johns Hopkins University Press.

Kimble, K. (2008). Psychiatric emergency issues in the general ed. *Emergency Nursing World*, 12–23.

Kleespies, P. M. (1998). *Emergencies in mental health practice*. New York, NY: Guilford Press.

Nadler-Moodie, M. (2010, May). Psychiatric emergencies in med-surg patients: Are you prepared? *American Nurse Today*, 7(4), 1–5.

Singh, J. P., Fazel, S., Gueorguieva, R., & Buchanan, A. (2014). Rates of violence in patients classified as high risk by structured risk assessment instruments. *The British Journal of Psychiatry*, 204(3), 180–187. doi: 10.1192/bjp.bp.113.131938

Stuart, G. (2009). *Principles and practice of psychiatric nursing* (9th ed.). St. Louis, MO: Mosby-Elsevier.

Swanson, J. W. (1994). Mental disorder, substance abuse, and community violence: An epidemiological approach. In J. Monahan & H. J. Steadman (Eds.), *Violence and mental disorder: Developments in risk assessment* (pp. 101–136). Chicago, IL: University of Chicago Press.

Tintinalli, J. E., Kelen, G. D., & Stapczynski, J. S. (2000). *Emergency medicine: A comprehensive study guide*. New York, NY: McGraw-Hill Professional Publishing.

Townsend, M. C. (2015). *Psychiatric mental health nursing: Concepts of care in evidence-based practice* (8th ed.). Philadelphia, PA: F. A. Davis Company.

Varcarolis, E. M. (2011). *Manual of psychiatric nursing care planning: Assessment guides, diagnoses, psychopharmacology* (4th ed.). New York, NY: Elsevier Health Sciences.

Vergare, M. J., Binder, R. L., Cook, I. A., Galanter, M., & Lu, F. G. (2006). *Practice guideline for the psychiatric evaluation of adults* (2nd ed.). Washington, DC: American Psychiatric Association.

Warren, E. (2009). Managing psychiatric emergencies. *Practice Nurse*, 37(2), 2–9.

PERFORMING A MENTAL STATUS ASSESSMENT

"Peace begins with a smile."
–Mother Teresa

OBJECTIVES

- Perform a legal status assessment
- Assess the patient's physical appearance
- Evaluate the patient's alertness, orientation, behavior, attitude, affect, and mood
- Analyze the patient's thought processes, thought content, attention, concentration, and memory
- Appraise the patient's judgment, insight, and intellect
- Note hallucinations and delusions
- Assess speech and motor activity
- Assess other issues to evaluate mental status
- Perform a risk assessment
- Formulate a de-escalation plan

New nurses often wonder when violence prevention *truly* begins. The answer is that it starts on the very first day a patient enters a healthcare facility, with a well-designed mental status assessment upon admission. This assessment gives healthcare professionals the information they need to safely care for the patient. It represents the single most important step in the clinical evaluation of an individual who suffers from or is suspected of having a mental disorder.

A mental status assessment is a person-to-person interview conducted by nursing staff as part of a comprehensive physical and psychosocial assessment. Conducting this assessment involves asking patients questions and noting their answers, while also making visual observations. The results of the assessment are recorded and documented in the patients' written or electronic health record and communicated in a unit report. In addition, findings are reported to the physician or psychiatrist in charge after admission for appropriate follow-up and intervention as needed.

> ☑ **NOTE** A strong clinical admission assessment is one of the most vital interventions to prevent healthcare violence (Singh, Fazel, Gueorguieva, & Buchanan, 2014).

Psychiatric facilities have long completed mental status and de-escalation assessments on all patients admitted to their facilities. In fact, The Joint Commission requires these assessments for mental health facilities. This is because many patients arrive at mental health facilities with a history of violence. Indeed, it's often the case that a patient's violent behavior is the reason for requiring treatment (Damon, Matthews, Sheehan, & Uebelacker, 2012). Recently, some healthcare facilities of other types have begun performing similar assessments to identify those at risk for escalation.

Mental status assessments may vary in their content. Generally speaking, however, a mental status assessment includes an evaluation of the patient's physical appearance; alertness, orientation, behavior, attitude, affect, and mood; thought processes, thought content, attention, concentration, and memory; judgment, insight, and intellect; whether the patient is experiencing hallucinations or delusions; and the patient's speech and motor activity (American Psychiatric Association [APA], 2013; Zuckerman, 2005). A mental status assessment might also involve evaluating a patient's legal status. Figure 10.1 shows a template for a standard mental status assessment.

Mental Status Assessment
_____

• Appearance:_____

• Mood:_____

• Affect:_____

• Speech:_____

• Motor Activity:_____

• Attention:_____

• Eye Contact:_____

• Concentration:_____

• Memory:_____

• Orientation:_____

• Cognition/Intellect:_____

• Insight Into Problems:_____

• Thought Process:_____

• Thought Content:_____

• Judgment:_____

• Hallucinations:_____

• Delusions:_____

FIGURE 10.1 A template for a standard mental status assessment.

In addition to the mental status assessment, nurses should conduct various risk assessments to determine the likelihood that the patient will hurt himself or someone else and work with the patient to formulate a de-escalation plan.

These assessments are founded in best practice and reflect established individual hospital policies for suicide assessment and violence prevention. Nursing staff can use the information obtained through the admission mental status assessment, risk assessments, and de-escalation plan assessment to determine risk and identify interventions to prevent harming behaviors and promote mental health, wellness, and recovery.

Violence prevention begins the first day a patient is admitted with an effective mental status and risk assessment (APA, 2013; Gately & Stabb, 2005; Haggård-Grann, Hallqvist, Långström, & Moller, 2006). A strong admission assessment is one of the most vital interventions to prevent healthcare violence (Singh et al., 2014).

> ☑ **NOTE** When performing a mental status assessment, you must also comply with all privacy guidelines as dictated by the Health Insurance Portability and Accountability Act (HIPAA) of 1996.

PERFORMING A LEGAL STATUS ASSESSMENT

Before you perform a mental status assessment, you must obtain legal consent from the patient. You should also evaluate and document the patient's legal status as part of the mental status assessment. Legal status refers to the following:

- The patient's age, marital status, and legal guardianship (if applicable) (Cazalas, 1979)

- Pending criminal charges or existing parole or probation issues

- Whether the patient's admission is voluntary or involuntary (court committed)

> ☑ **NOTE** Determining whether the patient's admission is voluntary or involuntary is vital to enable nurses to provide adequate, safe, and legal care as required by state laws.

ASSESSING THE PATIENT'S PHYSICAL APPEARANCE

Upon initial examination, as the admitting nurse, you should observe and document the appropriateness (or inappropriateness) of the patient's personal appearance. This means assessing the patient's apparel, including its condition and cleanliness. You should also evaluate personal hygiene and grooming—for example, whether the patient has dirty fingernails or emits body odor. It is particularly important to document observations that might indicate neglect (including self-neglect) or abuse. When documenting your observations, use specific and descriptive terms, such as meticulous, tasteful, conservative, bizarre, naked, disheveled, dirty, and so on (Hersen & Turner, 1987).

> ❓ **TIP** Use specific and descriptive terms when documenting your observations of the patient.

EVALUATING ALERTNESS, ORIENTATION, BEHAVIOR, ATTITUDE, AFFECT, AND MOOD

In addition to assessing a patient's physical appearance, you should evaluate and document demeanor, including alertness, disorientation, behavior, attitude, affect, and mood.

To assess patient alertness, observe whether the patient can keep awake and respond appropriately to questions. When documenting your observations, use words like confused, distracted, responsive, unresponsive, and so on to describe the patient's behavior (Lukas, 1993).

An orientation assessment enables you to determine the extent of the patient's association with reality or confusion (if any). To evaluate, ask the patient to state the present day, month, or year, or the place or present situation. Document your findings by using phrases like *oriented to time*, *oriented to place*, or *oriented to present situation*, or as *disoriented* (Zuckerman, 2005).

Evaluating the patient's behavior and attitude comes next. When documenting your observations, you can use any number of terms to describe this. These might include the following:

- **Combative behavior.** This describes behavior in which the patient strikes out at others.

- **Attention-seeking behavior.** This describes behavior in which the patient frequently makes unnecessary requests.

- **Ritualistic behavior.** This describes behavior in which the patient demonstrates repeated ritual behavior.

- **Decreased motivation and/or energy.** This describes behavior that demonstrates a lack of will or desire to participate in the everyday activities of daily living, leaving the patient appearing listless and depressed.

- **Staff-splitting behavior.** This describes behavior in which the patient attempts to cause conflict among staff.

- **Dependent behavior.** This describes behavior in which the patient asks others to complete tasks despite being able to complete the tasks independently (Sommers-Flanagan & Sommers-Flanagan, 1993).

- **Repetitive behavior.** This describes behavior in which the patient continuously repeats certain behaviors.

- **Isolative or withdrawn behavior.** This describes behavior in which the patient avoids social contact.

Table 10.1 offers suggestions for additional behavioral descriptors.

TABLE 10.1 Suggested Terms to Describe Behavior and Attitude

Normal or appropriate	Hostile	Aggressive	Agitated
Naïve	Docile	Suspicious	Evasive
Negative	Calm	Defensive	Threatening
Argumentative	Impulsive	Uncooperative	Splitting
Oppositional	Verbally or physically disruptive	Combative	Restless
Cooperative	Resistive	Dependent	Attention-seeking
Teary	Intrusive	Manipulative	Subject to explosive outbursts of anger

In addition to other aspects of the patient's demeanor, you should assess the patient's *affect*—in other words, a patient's capacity to vary outward expression of emotion. Affect fluctuates with changes in thought content and can be observed in the patient's facial expression, voice, and gestures.

Affect is often described in terms of quality (tone), quantity, range, and appropriateness. Common descriptors for affect include anxious, angry, irritable, and tearful. Other descriptors include the following:

- **Anhedonic.** The patient shows an inability to experience pleasure.

- **Apathetic.** The patient appears indifferent or shows an absence of emotion.

- **Flat.** The patient lacks signs of affective expression of emotion (Cook & Fontaine, 1991).

- **Blunted.** The patient displays a diminished intensity of emotion (Townsend, 2015).

- **Constricted.** The patient displays a diminished range of emotion.

- **Stable.** The patient displays a normal and consistent affect without sudden or unprovoked change.

- **Elated or elevated.** The patient seems more cheerful than normal.

- **Depressed.** The patient shows a diminished interest in everyday life, has a sad facial expression or teary eyes, has limited body movement, and voices feelings of sadness or despondency.

- **Full affect.** The patient shows a complete range of emotional expression.

- **Labile.** The patient shows repeated rapid shifts in emotion or affect.

- **Congruent.** The patient's behavior matches his or her mood.

- **Incongruent.** The patient's behavior does not match his or her mood.

Mood is defined as pervasive and sustained emotion that, in the extreme, can mark a person's perception of the world. Terms to describe mood include the following (APA, 2013):

- **Appropriate or euthymic.** The patient shows the normal mood for the current time and situation.

- **Apathetic.** The patient appears indifferent or uncaring.

- **Angry.** The patient behaves in a menacing way.

- **Depressed.** The patient is gloomy or sad.

- **Anxious.** The patient is uneasy, apprehensive, or worried.

- **Irritable.** The patient is ill-tempered or easily annoyed.

- **Dysphoric.** The patient shows an unpleasant mood, such as depression, anxiety, or irritability.

- **Fearful.** The patient shows a feeling of disquiet caused by awareness or expectation of danger.

- **Elevated.** The patient appears more cheerful than normal.

- **Euphoric.** The patient shows an exaggerated feeling of well-being.

- **Labile.** The patient shows repeated and rapid shifts in mood.

- **Rapid mood swing.** The patient shows a sudden or swift change in mood.

ANALYZING THOUGHT PROCESSES, THOUGHT CONTENT, ATTENTION, CONCENTRATION, AND MEMORY

An important part of any mental status assessment is an evaluation and documentation of the patient's thought processes, thought content, attention, concentration, and memory.

Terms to describe a patient's thought process include the following:

- **Logical or coherent.** The patient's communication shows consistency in reasoning and an easily understood thought process.

- **Blocked.** The patient cannot complete a train of thought.

- **Tangential.** The patient abruptly changes the topic of conversation.

- **Rambling.** The patient aimlessly wanders from topic to topic.

- **Circumstantial.** The patient provides unnecessary and tedious details and never gets to the point.

- **Clang association.** The patient incorrectly uses words that rhyme or sound alike (Sadock, Sadock, & Ruiz, 2015).

- **Depersonalized.** The patient seems detached from his or her own mind or body.

- **Perseveration.** The patient persistently repeats words, ideas, or subjects.

- **Flight of ideas.** The patient displays a continuous flow of accelerated speech and abruptly changes from topic to topic.

- **Loose association.** The patient communicates a series of seemingly unrelated thoughts.

- **Word salad or schizophasia.** The patient communicates a series of illogical word groupings that represent an extreme form of loose association (Cook & Fontaine, 1991).

- **Indecisive.** The patient is unable to make a decision.

> **? TIP** As you assess the patient's thought processes, pay special attention to problem-solving abilities. This will help you determine the person's ability to appropriately interpret external events.

While interacting with the patient, you should also evaluate thought content. Table 10.2 lists terms to describe thought content (Hersen & Turner, 1987).

TABLE 10.2 Suggested Terms to Describe Thought Content

Unremarkable	Forgetful	Appropriate
Coherent	Phobia or fears	Slow thought processes
Obsessive ideas	Ideas of harm	Feelings of unreality
Compulsions	Feelings of worthlessness	Persecution
Somatic complaints	Guilt	Sexual preoccupation
Hopelessness	Religiosity	Paranoid

> ☑ **NOTE** Somatic complaints are assessed and documented as part of the mental status assessment. The term *somatic complaint* describes psychological distress that is manifested as physical symptoms.

Attention and concentration are documented in the mental status assessment as good, fair, or poor. Memory should be documented as intact, confused, distracted, or amnesia. Memory status should also be documented. *Memory status* refers to one's ability to recall pertinent sensory-derived information from the four spheres of memory, which are as follows:

- **Immediate.** Immediate memory describes one's memory of information received in the immediate past.

- **Short-term.** Short-term memory is one's memory of information received today.

- **Recent.** Recent memory is one's memory of information received yesterday or in the recent past.

- **Remote (long-term).** Remote or long-term memory is one's memory of information given years ago.

All four of these spheres should be assessed and documented as good, fair, or poor. Finally, observations of confabulation should be documented. *Confabulation* is when someone creates a plausible but imaginary memory as a substitute for memory gaps (Boyd, 2008).

APPRAISING JUDGMENT, INSIGHT, AND INTELLECT

Insight and judgment are related concepts. *Insight* describes when you are aware of your own thoughts and emotions and can compare them with the thoughts and emotions of others (Haggård-Grann et al., 2006). Insight may be documented as moderate, little or none, excellent, or unrealistic (Zuckerman, 2005).

Judgment can be described as the ability to evaluate evidence to make a considered decision or arrive at a sensible conclusion. A patient's judgment is assessed and described as good, fair, or poor. Personal and social judgment skills are described in the same terms. In addition to evaluating the patient's judgment, you should gauge *impulsivity*—in other words, the patient's tendency to act without considering the consequences of the action.

Assessing the patient's intellect or cognitive abilities involves describing executive functions such as abstract reasoning and comprehension. Intellect is assessed and documented as being average, above average, below average, or concrete (Sommers-Flanagan & Sommers-Flanagan, 1993). To evaluate the patient's intellect, you can read the patient a proverb to interpret, such as "A rolling stone gathers no moss." Concrete intellect assessment involves determining whether the patient interprets the phrase in literal terms as it is spoken.

NOTING HALLUCINATIONS AND DELUSIONS

Hallucinations are false perceptions or perceptual experiences that occur in the absence of external stimuli (Boyd, 2008; Sommers-Flanagan & Sommers-Flanagan, 1993). To assess whether the patient is experiencing hallucinations, ask, "Do you ever see, hear, feel, smell, or taste something that is not actually there?" Terms to describe hallucinations for the purposes of documentation include the following:

- **Auditory.** The patient hears sounds or voices that are not actually present or real.

- **Visual.** The patient sees things that are not present or real.

- **Olfactory.** The patient smells something that is not present or real.

- **Tactile.** The patient feels sensations on the skin that are not present or real.

- **Gustatory.** The patient tastes something that is not present or real.

If the patient reports experiencing hallucinations, further questions are needed. For example, if the patient reports hearing voices, ask, "What are the voices saying?" to determine the content and intensity of the hallucination and whether safety precautions are called for.

Delusions are beliefs that have no basis in reality and that cannot be changed even in the face of evidence or logical reasoning (Kneisl & Trigoboff, 2009). An example of a delusion is an alert adult patient stating emphatically, "I am a Power Ranger!" If no delusions are present, you can simply mark none. But if the patient does appear delusional, you must document its type (see the following list) and include a narrative description of the delusional content.

- **Delusion of perception.** Patients believe they are being tormented, followed, tricked, or spied upon.

- **Delusion of grandeur.** Patients believe they personify greatness— for example, are famous or a god.

- **Reference delusion.** Patients believe that passages in books or magazines or scenes in a TV show or movie are about them (Kneisl & Trigoboff, 2009).

- **Influence delusion.** Patients believe that they are being compelled or controlled by others.

- **Somatic delusion.** Patients believe they are hopelessly ill when in fact no physical illness is present.

- **Religious delusion.** Patients express obsessive false beliefs of a religious nature. An example of this would be if they arrived in the unit with Bible verses glued to every inch of their body and yelled, "I have to wear these every day or God will destroy the planet!"

ASSESSING SPEECH AND MOTOR ACTIVITY

Speech provides clues into the patient's thought patterns, emotional patterns, and the presence of organization in cognitive function. Terms to describe a patient's speech include the following:

- **Confabulation.** The patient fabricates facts and events in response to events not remembered.

- **Ecolalia.** The patient repeats or echoes another's words (Boyd, 2008).

- **Loud.** The patient speaks in a high volume and with intensity.

- **Pressured.** The patient speaks quickly and loudly and is difficult to interrupt.

- **Soft.** The patient uses a pleasant, calm, and smooth voice.

- **Overproductive.** The patient speaks more than is necessary given the content of the conversation.

- **Underproductive or poverty of speech.** The patient speaks less than is necessary given the content of the conversation. This is conveyed through short replies to questions and seemingly reflects an inner emptiness.

- **Slurred speech.** The patient has difficulty pronouncing words (Sadock et al., 2015).

- **Mutism.** The patient is unable or unwilling to speak.

- **Stammering.** The patient's speech contains involuntary pauses and repetitions of sounds.

As with speech, alterations in motor activity (including gait) can provide clues into the patient's condition—in this case, whether the patient might be suffering from depression, organic disease, or other functional impairment. It can also provide indications of mental processes and the patient's mental status. Terms to describe a patient's motor activity include the following:

- **Normal.** The patient shows appropriate movement and range of motion.

- **Catatonic.** The patient appears to be in a state of stupor or excitement.

- **Echopraxia.** The patient imitates the body movements of another person.

- **Overactive.** The patient displays hyperactive movement (Hersen & Turner, 1987).

- **Psychomotor retardation.** The patient displays diminished movement.

- **Tremor.** The patient's limbs or extremities shake involuntarily.

- **Posturing.** The patient's extremities are rigid in a fixed position.

- **Tics.** The patient experiences spasmodic muscle contractions in the face or extremities.

- **Ataxic gait.** The patient displays poor coordination when moving extremities.

- **Repetitive acts.** The patient repeatedly and voluntarily moves extremities.

- **Agitated motor activity.** The patient's extremities move swiftly and abruptly.

- **Restless.** The patient displays constant shifting movement.

- **Involuntary movement.** The patient moves extremities involuntarily.

ADDITIONAL MENTAL STATUS ASSESSMENTS

In addition to the mental status assessments discussed, the patient should be asked about the following issues upon admission:

- Sleep disturbances such as insomnia or oversleeping

- Appetite disturbances such as loss of appetite

- Unintentional weight loss

- Nutritional status such as starvation and vitamin deficiencies

- Family history of mental illness

- History of substance abuse

- History of physical and sexual abuse

- History of self-harm

- History of violence

- Previous psychiatric hospitalizations

In addition, the patient's level of compliance with regard to medication should be assessed (Hersen & Turner, 1987). All these can provide insight into how likely it is a patient could experience aberrant, agitated, or aggressive behavior.

PERFORMING A RISK ASSESSMENT

A risk assessment is an essential part of mental health admissions and ongoing nursing care. Included in the risk assessment is an evaluation of the patient's suicidal and homicidal ideation—that is, whether the patient is a danger to himself or to others (McKnight, 2011) and if so the degree of lethality of intent (Abderhalden et al., 2008; Hersen & Turner, 1987; Zuckerman, 2005).

As part of the risk assessment, you should work with the patient to formulate a de-escalation plan to prevent harming behaviors during a hospital stay.

> ☑ **NOTE** Risk assessments increase staff awareness and ability to anticipate and potentially prevent aggression and violence (Hamrin, Iennaco, & Olsen, 2009; Johnson & Delaney, 2007).

The Joint Commission mandates that risk assessments be completed for all mental health facility inpatients deemed at risk to themselves or others within 24 hours of admission to prevent harming behaviors (The Joint Commission, 2008). Early risk assessment—especially on admission—enables the development of nursing interventions to negate harm toward self or others and promote improvement in mental health. Figure 10.2 outlines a sample risk-assessment procedure.

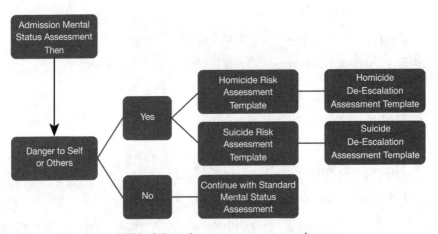

FIGURE 10.2 Risk-assessment procedure.

> ☑ **NOTE** Harming behaviors toward self or others are commitment criteria for both voluntary and involuntary treatment in every state.

As mentioned, one aspect of the risk assessment is determining whether the patient is suicidal. Suicide is seen as anger turned inward to the self. To gauge whether a patient is suicidal, ask whether there is an experience of suicidal thoughts. If the answer is yes, ask these follow-up questions and document the patient's answers. (Figure 10.3 shows a template that can be used to take down this information.)

- **Do you have a plan to harm yourself?** Having a plan to harm oneself is cause for alarm.

- **How are you planning to harm yourself?** This is to determine whether the patient has devised a *specific* plan to harm himself.

- **Do you really intend to harm yourself, or are these passive thoughts that you will not act on?** This is to gauge how seriously the patient intends self-harm.

- **Do you have a means to harm yourself available to you?** This refers to whether the patient has a weapon or instrument of suicide available.

☐ Suicidal Thoughts _____

☐ Suicidal Plan _____

☐ Suicidal Intent _____

☐ Suicidal Means _____

FIGURE 10.3 A template for assessing suicidal ideation.

☑ **NOTE** Seven out of every 100 people with depression go on to complete suicide, and two-thirds of people who successfully complete suicide were depressed at the time of their death. According to the American Association of Suicidology, the risk of suicide for people with major depression is 20 times greater than for the general population (2010). Finally, the lifetime risk of suicide for people with untreated depression is 20%.

You must also know the indicators of suicidal intent to prevent suicide. These indicators are conspicuous. One indicator is feelings of overwhelming anxiety. This is a major predisposing trigger for a suicide attempt. Another indicator is when a suicidal individual suddenly gives away valuable property and treasured belongings. Still another is when a severely depressed patient's outlook suddenly seems "better." This may indicate that the patient has made a decision and has the means for a successful suicide (Boyd, 2008; deSa & Price, 2007). Finally, a suicidal person might begin telephoning or texting others to say goodbye or write a suicide note as a farewell gesture.

Any assessment of a suicidal patient is multifaceted. It involves the following actions:

- Identifying existing risk factors such as financial stressors or recent losses

- Ascertaining whether the patient has ever attempted suicide in the past

- Determining whether the patient is experiencing suicidal thoughts

> **! CAUTION** Take all suicide threats seriously—including thoughts of suicide. If suicidal thoughts are present, ask the person if there is a plan, time, or location for a suicide attempt.

- Establishing whether the patient has the means available to commit suicide

- Examining whether the patient exhibits suicidal intent and has considered the likelihood of rescue (Saluja et al., 2004; Snow, Lascher, & Mottur-Pilson, 2000)

- Verifying whether the patient has made final arrangements—an indicator of serious intent to harm oneself

- Evaluating whether the patient is experiencing symptoms of depression

- Finding out if the patient has been abusing alcohol or drugs

- Seeing if the patient has displayed a tendency to isolate himself or to withdraw from family, friends, or the community

- Assessing the patient's mental status, including disorientation, disorganization, and anxiety level

- Exploring the patient's lifestyle and activities of daily living (e.g., whether the patient is homeless, uses a wheelchair, etc.)

- Detecting the presence of hostility

It's also important to assess protective factors such as the presence of a supportive significant other or family members to gauge the ability of the patient to resist stressors (U.S. Preventive Services Task Force, 2002).

Nurses must listen closely to determine whether a patient describes or mentions self-harm. If a patient says, "Yes, I am thinking about suicide now," the nurse must not leave the patient unobserved and must institute suicide precautions as indicated by the facility protocols. A one-to-one should be immediately initiated for safety, with one nurse observing the patient continuously to prevent self-harm until further evaluation is completed by a psychiatrist, physician, or mental health professional.

> ☑ **NOTE** It is especially important that an assessment of suicidal ideation and harmful intent toward self or others be completed as part of the mental status assessment.

As part of a risk assessment, in addition to assessing whether the patient is suicidal, you must determine whether there is intent to harm others—in other words, an intention to be violent or homicidal. Violent or homicidal ideation is less frequent than suicidal ideation, but it does happen. Detecting violent or homicidal ideation involves asking the same basic questions as you did to detect suicidal ideation, but geared toward harming others rather than the self:

- Do you have a plan to harm others?

- How are you planning to harm others?

- Do you really intend to harm others, or are these passive thoughts that you will not act on?

- Do you have a means to harm others available?

Figure 10.4 shows a template you can use to assess homicidal ideation.

☐ Homicidal Thoughts _____
☐ Homicidal Plan _____
☐ Homicidal Intent _____
☐ Homicidal Means _____

FIGURE 10.4 A template for assessing homicidal ideation.

Signs and symptoms of violent or homicidal intent include the following:

- A lack of remorse or empathy for others
- Low tolerance for boredom
- Impulsivity
- The presence of significant stressors
- The recent loss (or threat of loss) of someone or something meaningful to the patient

Additional indicators include delusions of persecution, threats of harm to others, existence of a plan to harm others, access to harmful weapons, history of violence, and a labile mood (Dubin & Weiss, 1997). Finally, access to a victim of choice may increase the likelihood of violence or homicide.

When assessing a violent patient, it is important to determine the seriousness of the risk of potential harm to others. Threats of violence are evaluated from general to specific threat risks. General risks include random thoughts of harm, such as the patient stating, "I feel like I want to throw something at someone." Specific threat risks are specific—for example, if a patient states an uncontrollable urge to harm a specific person, as well as a plan, weapon, time, and location. Whether the risk is imminent should also be assessed.

When assessing the patient, the nurse must listen carefully. If the patient states the intent to harm someone, the nurse must ensure safety of self and institute assaultive precautions as per facility protocols.

If you determine a patient might be violent (toward the self or toward others), you should also expand the risk assessment to identify possible triggers. This is called an *admission risk assessment*. This assessment assists in identifying precursors to violence to prevent it from coming to pass until the patient regains emotional stability (Chabora, Judge-Gorny, & Grogan, 2003). Figure 10.5 contains a sample admission risk assessment questionnaire based on Joint Commission recommendations that you can use as a template. You can use the patient's answers in this assessment to develop specific treatment and management plans to reduce the risk of violence (Allen, 2000).

> ☑ **NOTE** To prevent violence, it is important to routinely assess, document, and monitor risk factors for assault and violence, starting with the initial investigation and continuing on an ongoing basis (Abderhalden et al., 2008; McKnight, 2011).

Do any of the following render you emotionally upset, stressed, or agitated/violent?

☐ Touch
☐ Shouting/Loud Noise
☐ Physical Force
☐ Restraints
☐ Derogatory Names
☐ Television
☐ Uniforms
☐ Crying
☐ Anger
☐ Isolation
☐ Threats
☐ Other _____

FIGURE 10.5 Admission risk assessment template.

FORMULATING A DE-ESCALATION PLAN

The Joint Commission requires that a de-escalation plan be completed for all mental health inpatients deemed a danger to themselves or others (The Joint Commission, 2008). Many medical facilities also use de-escalation plans to prevent healthcare violence in general. This plan should be completed upon admission as part of a comprehensive mental health assessment (McKnight, 2011; Singh, Grann, Lichtenstein, Långström, & Fazel, 2012).

> ☑ **NOTE** In the case of electronic mental health risk assessments, if the patient requires completion of either the homicide or the suicide risk assessment, screens with steps to develop a de-escalation plan will appear automatically during the patient interview.

You complete this plan in collaboration with the patient. This involves performing a de-escalation assessment to obtain information from the patient about which types of interventions will be most effective in promoting calm in the event of agitation or depression to prevent violence or self-harm (Agency for Healthcare Research and Quality, 2007; American Psychiatric Association,

American Psychiatric Nurses Association, & National Association of Psychiatric Health Systems, 2007). The assessment also identifies events or experiences that may cause the patient to become upset (also called triggers) (Chabora et al., 2003; Jeffrey & Austen, 2005). Figure 10.6 shows a sample de-escalation plan assessment (McKnight, 2011). This assessment is based on Joint Commission standard requirements.

Do any of the following activities assist you to calm when under stress?

☐ Television
☐ Going for Walk
☐ Deep Breathing Exercises
☐ Puzzles/Games
☐ Time Alone/Quiet Time
☐ Physical Activity
☐ Speaking to Family, Friends, or Healthcare Staff
☐ Reading Book, Bible, or Magazine
☐ Taking Nap
☐ Music
☐ Warm Blanket
☐ Other _____

FIGURE 10.6 A sample de-escalation plan assessment.

✅ **NOTE** The best de-escalation interventions are individualized and originate from the patient. The assessing professional determines and documents which de-escalation intervention the patient prefers during the mental status assessment. This information becomes a permanent part of the mental status assessment.

RISK ASSESSMENT

Mr. Sawyer is a 43-year-old well-nourished man admitted voluntarily to a behavioral health facility for complaints of depressed mood lasting over one year. Mr. Sawyer has a history of previous admissions and was discharged two months ago with a diagnosis of major depression. Mr. Sawyer was previously stabilized on *escitalopram* 10 mg daily. During questioning, Mr. Sawyer states that he stopped taking his prescribed *escitalopram* two weeks ago and has begun feeling "down and depressed." Mr. Sawyer arrived at the facility from a local emergency department and appears sad and despondent.

An extensive mental status assessment was completed on Mr. Sawyer upon admission. This included a risk assessment. Based on information provided by the patient upon admission (at which time he verbally threatened self-harm and suicidal intent), and on information obtained from the patient's history, lab results, and the emergency department staff, the patient was deemed a danger to himself.

The admitting nurse completes a suicide risk assessment by asking the patient a series of questions. To document the patient's answers, the nurse uses a suicide risk template designed for this explicit purpose (refer to Figure 10.3). The questions and answers are as follows:

- **Are you experiencing suicidal thoughts?** Mr. Sawyer says that he is experiencing constant thoughts of suicide.

- **Do you have a plan to commit suicide?** Mr. Sawyer says that he plans to use a weapon such as a knife to commit suicide.

- **How serious is your intent to harm yourself?** Mr. Sawyer says that he intends to harm himself when he returns home.

- **Do you have the means by which to harm yourself?** Mr. Sawyer says that he has a weapon hidden at home.

All four questions in the suicide risk template are checked as positive for Mr. Sawyer, as he has thoughts, a plan, intent, and a means to attempt self-harm. The degree of lethality or intent to do harm is also determined, documented, and reported to the psychiatrist and physician responsible for initiating precautions to prevent self-harm.

Because Mr. Sawyer is at risk for self-harm, a de-escalation plan is also completed. When questioned about de-escalation preferences, Mr. Sawyer states that watching television is the only technique that helps him calm down when he feels the urge to self-harm. Mr. Sawyer is also assessed for events or experiences that trigger an agitated state. He states that loud noises agitate him. The de-escalation interventions and triggers identified in the assessment are documented in the electronic health record and placed in the unit report.

Performing the admission mental status assessment and completing the de-escalation plan prevents Mr. Sawyer from self-harm and makes the healthcare unit safe for everyone.

REFERENCES

Abderhalden, C., Needham, I., Dassen, T., Halfens, R., Haug, H. J., & Fischer, J. E. (2008). Structured risk assessment and violence in acute psychiatric wards: Randomised controlled trial. *British Journal of Psychiatry: The Journal of Mental Science, 193*(1), 44–50. doi: 10.1192/bjp.bp.107.045534

Agency for Healthcare Research and Quality. (2007). *Roadmap to seclusion and restraint free mental health services.* Retrieved from https://innovations.ahrq.gov/qualitytools/roadmap-seclusion-and-restraint-free-mental-health-services

Allen, M. H. (2000). Managing the agitated psychotic patient: A reappraisal of the evidence. *The Journal of Clinical Psychiatry, 61*(Suppl 14), 11–21.

American Association of Suicidology. (2010). Some facts about suicide and depression. *American Association of Suicidology.* Retrieved from https://www.dartmouth.edu/~eap/library/depressionandsuicide.pdf

American Psychiatric Association. (2013). *Diagnostic and statistical manual of mental disorders (DSM-5).* Washington, DC: American Psychiatric Association.

American Psychiatric Association, American Psychiatric Nurses Association, & National Association of Psychiatric Health Systems. (2007). *Learning from each other: Success stories and ideas for reducing restraint/seclusion in behavioral health.* Retrieved from http://www.restraintfreeworld.org/documents/Learning%20From%20Each%20Other.pdf

Boyd, M. A. (2008). *Psychiatric nursing: Contemporary practice* (4th ed.). Philadelphia, PA: Lippincott, Williams & Wilkins.

Cazalas, M. W. (1979). *Nursing and the law* (3rd ed.). Germantown, MD: Aspen Systems Corporation.

Chabora, N., Judge-Gorny, M., & Grogan, K. (2003). The Four S Model in Action for de-escalation: An innovative state hospital-university collaborative endeavor. *Journal of Psychosocial Nursing and Mental Health Services, 41*(1), 22–28.

Cook, S., & Fontaine, K. (1991). *Essentials of mental health nursing* (2nd ed.). Redwood City, CA: Addison-Wesley Nursing.

Damon, L., Matthews, J., Sheehan, J., & Uebelacker, L. (2012). *Inpatient psychiatric nursing: Clinical strategies & practical interventions.* New York, NY: Springer Publishing Company.

deSa, P., & Price, D. W. (2007). Diagnosis and treatment of major depression 2007. *The Permanente Journal, 11*(3), 35–42.

Dubin, W., & Weiss, K. (1997). *Handbook of psychiatric emergencies.* Torrance, CA: Homestead School.

Gately, L. A., & Stabb, S. D. (2005). Psychology students' training in the management of potentially violent clients. *Professional Psychology: Research and Practice, 36*(6), 681–687.

Haggård-Grann, U., Hallqvist, J., Långström, N., & Möller, J. (2006). Short-term effects of psychiatric symptoms and interpersonal stressors on criminal violence: A case-crossover study. *Social Psychiatry and Psychiatric Epidemiology, 41*(7), 532–540.

Hamrin, V., Iennaco, J., & Olsen, D. (2009). A review of ecological factors affecting inpatient psychiatric unit violence: Implications for relational and unit cultural improvements. *Issues in Mental Health Nursing, 30*(4), 214–226. doi: 10.1080/01612840802701083

Hersen, M., & Turner, S. M. (1987). *Diagnostic interviewing.* New York, NY: Plenum Press.

Jeffrey, D., & Austen, S. (2005). Adapting de-escalation techniques with deaf service users. *Nursing Standard, 19*(49), 41–47.

Johnson, M. E., & Delaney, K. R. (2007). Keeping the unit safe: The anatomy of escalation. *Journal of the American Psychiatric Nurses Association, 13*(1), 42–50.

The Joint Commission. (2008). *2008 comprehensive accreditation manual for hospitals: The official handbook.* Oak Brook, IL: Joint Commission Resources.

Kneisl, C. R., & Trigoboff, E. (2009). *Contemporary psychiatric-mental health nursing* (2nd ed.). Upper Saddle River, NJ: Prentice Hall.

Lukas, S. (1993). *Where to start and what to ask: An assessment handbook.* New York, NY: W. W. Norton & Company.

McKnight, S. (2011). Risk assessment in the electronic age: Application of the circle of caring model. *Online Journal of Nursing Informatics, 15*(3).

Sadock, B. J., Sadock, V. A., & Ruiz, P. (2015). *Kaplan and Sadock's synopsis of psychiatry: Behavioral sciences/clinical psychiatry* (11th ed.). New York, NY: Lippincott, Williams & Wilkins.

Saluja, G., Iachan, R., Scheidt, P. C., Overpeck, M. D., Sun, W., & Giedd, J. N. (2004). Prevalence of and risk factors for depressive symptoms among young adolescents. *Archives of Pediatrics and Adolescent Medicine, 158*(8), 760–765.

Singh, J. P., Fazel, S., Gueorguieva, R., & Buchanan, A. (2014). Rates of violence in patients classified as high risk by structured risk assessment instruments. *The British Journal of Psychiatry, 204*(3), 180–187. doi: 10.1192/bjp.bp.113.131938

Singh, J. P., Grann, M., Lichtenstein, P., Långström, N., & Fazel, S. (2012). A novel approach to determining violence risk in schizophrenia: Developing a stepped strategy in 13,806 discharged patients. *PLOS ONE, 7*(2), e31727. doi: 10.1371/journal.pone.0031727

Snow, V., Lascher, S., & Mottur-Pilson, C. (2000). Pharmacologic treatment of acute major depression and dysthymia. *Annals of Internal Medicine, 132*(9), 738–742.

Sommers-Flanagan, J., & Sommers-Flanagan, R. (1993). *Foundations of therapeutic interviewing.* Boston, MA: Allyn & Bacon.

Townsend, M. C. (2015). *Psychiatric mental health nursing: Concepts of care in evidence-based practice* (8th ed.). Philadelphia, PA: F. A. Davis Company.

U.S. Preventive Services Task Force. (2002). Screening for depression: Recommendations and rationale. *Annals of Internal Medicine, 136*(10), 760–764.

Zuckerman, E. L. (2005). *Clinician's thesaurus: The guide to conducting interviews and writing psychological reports* (6th ed.). New York, NY: The Guilford Press.

11

DE-ESCALATION OF PATIENTS WITH MENTAL DISORDERS

"Peace is its own reward."
–Mahatma Gandhi

OBJECTIVES

- Discover the four most commonly treated mental disorders

- Find out how to identify patients suffering from schizophrenia, bipolar disorder, major depressive disorder, and panic disorder

- Explore how to assess patients suffering from schizophrenia, bipolar disorder, major depressive disorder, and panic disorder

- See how to de-escalate patients suffering from schizophrenia, bipolar disorder, major depressive disorder, and panic disorder

- Compare identification, assessment, and de-escalation practices for the four disorders

Healthcare facilities frequently treat patients for concerns related to four promi-nent mental disorders: schizophrenia, bipolar disorder, major depressive disorder, and panic disorder. Although these disorders are mental in nature, individuals who suffer from them are frequently treated on an outpatient basis in clinics, hospitals, and extended care facilities. Often these individuals are hospitalized for physical health issues that exacerbate their mental health condition.

Schizophrenia, bipolar disorder, major depressive disorder, and panic disorder are all very different conditions, with their own unique manifestations. When a patient suffering from one of these disorders seeks treatment, it's critical to use assessment and interventional techniques that are appropriate for that indi-vidual's disorder to prevent escalation and ensure proper patient-centered care. That's the focus of this chapter.

ASSESSING AND DE-ESCALATING PATIENTS WITH SCHIZOPHRENIA

Schizophrenia refers to a group of severe disabling psychiatric disorders marked by a withdrawal from reality. Schizophrenia is characterized by severe emotional, behavioral, or intellectual disturbances. Symptoms of schizophrenia include dis-torted perceptions of reality, diminished ability to think rationally, and impaired emotional experience and social engagement (American Psychiatric Association [APA], 2013; Minzenberg, Yoon, & Carter, 2011). Other signs and symptoms of schizophrenia are disorganized thoughts and behaviors, negative mood states, and behavioral impulsivity. Finally, people who suffer from schizophrenia may at times experience delusions and hallucinations. Auditory hallucinations—hearing "voices"—are common in schizophrenia.

> ☑ **NOTE** Schizophrenia is a serious and pervasive lifelong mental disorder. It is present in 1% of the population and affects males and females in equal numbers. Between 5% and 6% of people with schizophrenia die by suicide (APA, 2013; Harris & Barraclough, 1999).

The treatment of schizophrenia involves a multidimensional and interdisciplin-ary approach. Treatment options include the following:

- **Psychopharmacology.** This includes antipsychotic medications to reduce or eliminate the auditory and visual hallucinations that often occur with schizophrenia.

- **Psychosocial treatment and rehabilitation.** This helps reintegrate individuals with schizophrenia into the family setting and broader community for holistic recovery.

- **Vocational counseling.** This assists people with schizophrenia by providing job training to gain employment or return to a vocation (Boyd, 2008; Kane, 2003).

- **Electroconvulsive therapy (ECT).** ECT involves applying an electric current to the brain through electrodes that are placed on the patient's temples to produce a grand mal seizure. ECT is used primarily for patients who are resistant to treatment with medication. Some individuals with treatment-resistant schizophrenia may be candidates for ECT.

When assessing patients who suffer from schizophrenia, you'll want to pay particular attention to whether they are experiencing an altered sensory-perceptual state or altered thought processes (such as delusions) or exhibiting aggressive behavior.

> **⚠ CAUTION** There is robust evidence that individuals who suffer from schizophrenia are at a higher risk of perpetrating violence toward others than the general population (Hodgins, 2008; Lehman et al., 2004).

You may be able to tell whether patients are experiencing an altered sensory-perceptual state simply by observing them. If patients adopt a listening pose, talk or laugh to themselves, or frequently stop talking mid-sentence, this could indicate they are experiencing such a state—in other words, hallucinating.

If you determine that patients are indeed hallucinating, convey an attitude of acceptance. Encourage them to share the contents of the hallucination with you. Ask them, "Are you hearing a voice talking in your head?" If the answer is yes, ask, "What is the voice saying?" Do not reinforce the hallucination, however. Use the term "the voice" instead of words like "it" or "they" that validate the notion that the voice is real. In a kind but respectful manner, tell the patients that you do not hear the voice. Say, "Although I know that the voice is very real to you, I do not hear any voices speaking." This presents reality to patients without challenging them.

> **? TIP** Try to connect the patient's experience of hallucinations to times of increased anxiety and stress to help the patient understand this relationship.

As with patients experiencing hallucinations, if you determine that patients are experiencing altered thought processes—in other words, are delusional—you should convey your acceptance of them as people but not of the delusion. Do not argue with patients about the delusion or aggressively deny their beliefs, however. Instead, use reasonable doubt as a therapeutic technique. For example, say, "I understand what you are saying, but it seems strange that your neighbor would want to pour poison in your yard."

Also assess for suicidal or homicidal ideation using the templates discussed in Chapter 10, "Performing a Mental Status Assessment." If indicated, complete a suicide risk assessment and take all necessary safety precautions.

To reduce incidences of anger with patients suffering from schizophrenia, try to limit how many staff members work with them. Interactions that encourage a one-to-one relationship are best. This helps promote the development of trusting relationships. Also, be honest with the patients and keep all promises. Finally, avoid laughing, joking, whispering, or talking quietly in front of patients such that they can see you but not hear what is being said (Jeffrey & Austen, 2005). Otherwise, the patients will likely grow suspicious, and their level of aggression could mount.

Here are additional tips for de-escalating patients who suffer from schizophrenia (or preventing escalation in the first place):

- Frequently observe the patient's behavior. Do this the same way you carry out routine activities to avoid causing the patient to grow suspicious (Gately & Stabb, 2005).

- Keep communications brief and simple.

- Maintain a matter-of-fact yet friendly approach and convey a calm attitude.

- Encourage the patient to verbalize any feelings of anxiety, tension, fear, or insecurity.

- Encourage the patient to engage in relaxation exercises such as deep breathing techniques to reduce anxiety.

- Encourage the patient to engage in thought-stopping techniques. *Thought-stopping* is the practice of identifying negative feelings and thoughts (e.g., an unpleasant memory of trauma), saying to yourself, "I will not allow that thought into my mind," and then engaging in a distracting, pleasant activity.

- Encourage the patient to engage in diversional activities.

- Find a physical outlet to redirect the patient and reduce the anxiety, such as physical exercise (Agency for Healthcare Research and Quality, 2007).

- Reorient the patient to reality. Talk to the patient about real events and real people. Discourage the patient from brooding on irrational thoughts (Hilgers, 2003; Hodgins, 2008).

- Remove environmental stimuli. For example, guide the patient away from crowded areas, eliminate loud noise, and dim the lights.

- Remove harmful objects from the patient's environment for safety.

- Avoid touching the patient without warning. Always ask the patient's permission first (Townsend, 2015).

- Administer medications as ordered by the provider. Monitor medication for its effectiveness and adverse side effects.

- Have sufficient staff available to assist if needed. Use the "buddy system" during all de-escalation interventions (Copeland & Henry, 2017).

TEST YOURSELF

SCHIZOPHRENIA Mr. Haley is a 26-year-old man who was diagnosed with schizophrenia two years ago. After dropping out of high school, Mr. Haley went to live with his grandparents in a neighboring state. Mr. Haley remained restless and was never able to truly establish any type of meaningful life or vocation. Mr. Haley never attempted to make friends and remained alienated from his parents and siblings.

Mr. Haley had frequent altercations with local law enforcement and spent several months in the county jail. When Mr. Haley was released from jail, he refused to return home to his grandparent's house. Instead, he became homeless and was living on the streets.

continues

A concerned social worker from a nearby church found Mr. Haley sitting on a street corner mumbling incoherently to himself and calling out to "voices" talking in his head. The social worker brought Mr. Haley to the emergency department to be evaluated.

Mr. Haley complains of seeing "demons" and makes little eye contact. He appears apathetic and answers questions by saying only "yes" or "no." Mr. Haley's hygiene is poor and his clothing is tattered. Mr. Haley's affect is blunted, and his speech is a soft monotone. Mr. Haley is responding strongly to internal stimuli.

How would you handle this situation?

ASSESSING AND DE-ESCALATING PATIENTS WITH BIPOLAR DISORDER

Bipolar disorder is a chronic mood disorder characterized by cycles of intense mood swings. Patients alternate between a manic state, in which they experience an exhilarating euphoria, and a depressed state, in which they experience intense depression. Interspersed between these two states are periods of normal mood and behavior.

> ✅ **NOTE** Bipolar disorder used to be called manic-depressive disorder.

Bipolar disorder affects 2.6% of the adult U.S. population. It affects males and females equally (APA, 2013; Townsend, 2015). There is a genetic link to bipolar disorder. It is an autosomal dominant disorder. People who have a first-degree relative who suffers from bipolar disorder have a 10-times greater risk of developing the disorder themselves.

Bipolar disorder can be effectively treated and managed with therapy and with medication such as lithium and valproic acid. The goals of care for bipolar disorder are stabilization of mood, improved self-control, better quality of life, and recovery from mental illness.

Symptoms of bipolar disorder vary depending on whether the patient is in a manic state or a depressive state. Table 11.1 lists common manic-state symptoms, and Table 11.2 lists common depressive-state symptoms.

TABLE 11.1 **Common Manic-State Symptoms**

Impulsivity	Inflated self-esteem	Insomnia
Grandiosity	Hyperirritability	Excessive pressured speech
Distractibility	Increased social activity	Psychomotor agitation
Participation in high-risk activities (promiscuity, compulsive shopping, unwise business investments, etc.)	Racing thoughts	Extreme euphoria

APA, 2013; Townsend, 2015

TABLE 11.2 **Common Depressive-State Symptoms**

Psychomotor agitation or psychomotor retardation	Fatigue	Inability to concentrate
Guilt	Recurrent thoughts of death	Feelings of sadness
Feelings of emptiness	Feelings of hopelessness	Feelings of worthlessness

APA, 2013; Townsend, 2015

> ✅ **NOTE** Manifestations of bipolar disorder often lead to severe psychosocial difficulties. These include alienation from friends, family, and coworkers; divorce; sexually transmitted diseases (STDs); job loss; the accumulation of debt; and problems with daily life (APA, 2013).

Some de-escalation interventions are appropriate for patients experiencing a manic episode, while others apply to patients in a depressed state. For example, if patients are experiencing a manic episode, it might help to involve them in activities that require gross motor movements to dissipate some of the energy associated with mania. When they become fatigued, suggest that they take a short daytime nap. In contrast, if patients are experiencing a depressed episode, provide positive reinforcement that the depression will lift. Also be alert for any signs of suicidal ideation. If indicated, complete a suicide risk assessment. (See Chapter 10 and take all necessary safety precautions.)

Other de-escalation interventions apply regardless of the patients' state. For example, it is important during both manic and depressed episodes to provide for their physical needs, such as nutrition, hydration, and rest. Encourage them to eat regular meals with adequate nutritional and fluid intake. If they are unable to address their own personal hygiene, assist if needed. Also monitor medication effects, levels, and side effects. As symptoms diminish, encourage increased self-care in all activities of daily living.

> **⚠ CAUTION** Patients with bipolar disorder can escalate quickly. Observe these patients frequently so you can intervene early if needed. Be alert for signs of escalating behaviors such as fist-clenching, verbal threats, and striking at objects.

Here are additional tips for de-escalating patients who suffer from bipolar disorder:

- Speak to patients in a calm, clear, and self-confident manner.
- Provide the patients with emotional support.
- Set realistic goals for appropriate behavior.
- Encourage patients to participate in diversional activities that require only a short attention span.
- Maintain a calm and quiet therapeutic environment with a low level of stimuli—few people, low noise, and dim light—to aid in calming. If needed, guide patients away from large groups, noxious noise, bright colors, or chaotic environments (Chabora, Judge-Gorny, & Grogan, 2003).
- Keep the environment free of hazardous items to prevent patients from harming themselves or others.
- Allow patients to speak to relieve their internal need for excessive verbalization.
- Listen attentively to patient requests with a neutral professional attitude.
- Set limits to counteract demanding, hyperactive, or manipulative behavior.
- Avoid power struggles.
- Provide consistent responses to aggressive, manipulative, or acting-out behavior (Townsend, 2015).
- Encourage patients to engage in relaxation exercises such as deep breathing to reduce stress.
- Remind patients that they are partners in the effort to maintain a safe environment, that they are responsible for controlling their own behavior, and

that aggressive or violent behavior such as threatening harm or striking out at others is not acceptable.

- Have sufficient staff available to assist if needed, and use the "buddy system" during all de-escalation interventions.

When patients regain self-control, conduct a debriefing to allow them to verbalize their feelings, determine the cause for the outburst, and generate suggestions to prevent future episodes.

TEST YOURSELF

BIPOLAR DISORDER Claire is a 20-year-old artist who lives alone in an apartment in New York. Claire was diagnosed with bipolar disorder at age 15. She was stabilized on lithium, which she took twice daily.

Claire completed high school and received an art scholarship from a prominent New York university. After moving to New York to attend university three weeks ago, Claire stated that she didn't like the way lithium made her mouth feel dry and stopped taking it.

After being off her medication for three weeks, Claire decided to participate in a local "Art in the Park" art show. During the art show, Claire stated that she no longer liked her paintings. Screaming, she smashed the paintings to the ground, breaking each one into pieces. Claire also attempted to smash the paintings of other nearby artists.

Law enforcement was called to the scene. Claire began running around the park, screaming. She fell over a table and fractured her right wrist. Law-enforcement officers brought Claire to the medical center for admission. The emergency department physician treating her fractured wrist has ordered a lithium level.

How would you handle this situation?

ASSESSING AND DE-ESCALATING PATIENTS WITH MAJOR DEPRESSIVE DISORDER

More than 9.5% of American adults suffer from major depressive disorder. The APA (2013) defines *major depressive disorder* as a condition in which someone experiences five prominent depressed symptoms during a two-week period that cause the person substantial distress. Table 11.3 lists possible symptoms.

TABLE 11.3 Depressive Symptoms

Depressed mood	Diminished interest or pleasure in all activities	Significant weight loss
Significant weight gain	Insomnia	Hypersomnia
Psychomotor agitation	Psychomotor retardation	Fatigue or loss of energy
Feelings of worthlessness	Excessive inappropriate guilt	Diminished ability to think or concentrate
Indecisiveness	Recurrent thoughts of death	Recurrent suicidal ideation

A suicide attempt or a specific plan for suicide is another symptom of major depressive disorder. Indeed, major depressive disorder is the psychiatric diagnosis most commonly associated with suicide. For information about assessing whether a patient is suicidal, see Chapter 10. If a patient is actively suicidal, initiate constant one-on-one observation—in which one nurse constantly monitors one patient—as per healthcare facility policy to prevent self-harm. Also implement the facility suicide prevention plan if one is available.

Effective de-escalation techniques are required for people who suffer from major depressive disorder for optimal recovery outcomes. One of the primary interventions for relief of depressive symptoms is to encourage the patient to verbalize (Gagné, Furman, Carpenter, & Price, 2000; Goldberg, 1998). Verbalizing will give the person a feeling of being heard and understood. It will also assist the nurse in developing therapeutic rapport with the patient.

Drawing Out a Depressive Patient

Communicating with a depressed patient is not an easy task. Many are reluctant to converse, preferring to remain silent. Here are some techniques to help you get the patient talking:

- Assume an active role in initiating communication. To begin, try sharing observations about the person's behavior—for example, "You're sitting here alone, looking sad. Is that how you feel?"

- Make eye contact.

- Speak slowly and allow adequate time for the person to respond.

- Listen attentively when the person is speaking, and don't interrupt.

- Maintain a nonjudgmental attitude.

- Avoid feigned cheerfulness, but don't hesitate to laugh with the person and to point out the value of humor.

- Encourage the person to write down all feelings (Karasu, Gelenberg, Wang, & Merriam, 2000).

Here are some other de-escalation techniques that are effective for patients who suffer from major depressive disorder:

- Encourage patients to socialize with friends or family to help lift their mood.

- Encourage patients to take spiritual measures to feel better—for example, reading the Bible or another religious text.

- Divert patients' attention by suggesting they read a magazine, watch TV, or listen to music.

- Remove harmful objects from the patients' environment (Boyd, 2008; Townsend, 2015).

- Teach the patients problem-solving skills.

- Educate the patients on positive coping skills for managing stress, such as diaphragmatic breathing, meditation, and yoga.

ASSESSING AND DE-ESCALATING PATIENTS WITH PANIC DISORDER

Anxiety is defined as an intense feeling of apprehension or uneasiness due to the perception of danger from an unknown source (Townsend, 2015). Experts identify four levels of anxiety:

- **Mild.** People with mild anxiety experience a sharpened ability to think, reason, and learn. Mild anxiety is not destabilizing. In fact, it can be beneficial, as people in a mild state of anxiety can learn more.

- **Moderate.** With moderate anxiety, the individual's focus begins to narrow until attention, perception, and problem-solving skills become impaired.

- **Severe.** In this state, the person experiences a markedly reduced ability to cope, very narrowed perception, an inability to concentrate, internally directed attention, severely reduced thinking, difficulty reasoning, and impaired problem-solving skills.

- **Panic.** At this level, the individual experiences extremely maladaptive responses to stressors, characterized by greatly impaired perception, complete disorganization of personality, and an inability to reason, solve problems, or even think coherently (Boyd, 2008). People experiencing panic-level anxiety become completely unable to function safely without assistance. In this state, people can become a danger to themselves or others.

A *panic disorder* is a type of anxiety disorder characterized by recurring episodes of sudden and intense fear and panic-level anxiety. The episodes develop swiftly, for no apparent reason and with no obvious precipitating event, and can trigger severe physical and emotional reactions, including intense fear, apprehension, and feelings of impending doom (APA, 2013; Tompkins, 2010). These episodes are called panic attacks.

> ✓ **NOTE** Between 2% and 3% of Americans and Europeans suffer from a panic disorder.

The APA (2013) *Diagnostic and Statistical Manual of Mental Disorders (DSM-5)* defines a *panic attack* as an abrupt surge of intense fear or discomfort. A panic attack reaches its peak within minutes and is short in duration—about 30 minutes. The regularity of panic attacks varies from frequent, short bursts to perhaps once a week (Edlund & Swann, 1987). During a panic attack, the person experiences four or more symptoms. Table 11.4 delineates these symptoms.

TABLE 11.4 Panic Attack Symptoms

Palpitations	Sweating	Trembling or shaking
Shortness of breath	A feeling of being smothered	A feeling of choking
Chest pain	Nausea	Abdominal discomfort
Dizziness	Unsteadiness	Light-headedness
Feeling faint	Feeling chills	Feeling hot
Paresthesia (numbness or tingling)	De-realization (feelings of unreality)	De-personalization
Fear of losing control	Fear of going crazy	Fear of dying

APA, 2013; Ballenger & Fyer, 1993

The assessment process for patients suffering from anxiety disorders begins upon their admission to a healthcare or mental health facility or on their first day of treatment. This assessment should cover the following:

- Whether the individual has suffered repeated panic attacks in the past (McGrandles & McCaig, 2013)

- What relieved the anxiety in past attacks

- Symptoms of the attack

- The duration and intensity of symptoms

- When symptoms first occurred

- A history of psychosocial stressors

- Ongoing conflicts that could be triggering the attacks

> **? TIP**   Identifying possible triggers may help the patient predict and prevent future panic attacks (Boyd, 2008; Pollard, Obermeier, & Cox, 1987).

With panic attacks, early intervention can lead to the quick and successful resolution of the anxiety and panic state. Here are key de-escalation techniques to keep in mind when dealing with patients experiencing a panic attack:

- Never leave them alone. Remain with them and reassure them that they are safe.

- Stay calm and serene (Sargent, 1990). Be a role model for the patients to emulate.

- Speak clearly and directly, and use as few words as possible.

- Avoid touching the patients until therapeutic rapport is established. Even then, ask permission first.

- Help the patients grasp the reality of their situation.

- Give directions one at a time. Make sure each direction is understood before proceeding to the next one.

- Reduce environmental stimuli (Tompkins, 2010). For example, eliminate noise or dim the lights (assuming the patients do not have vision or gait problems).

- Provide a safe environment to protect the patients and others from harm.

- Allow the patients to pace, and walk with them. Walking (or other physical exercise) helps expend some of the energy generated during a panic state.

- Encourage the patients to verbalize their feelings and to express their emotions freely.

- Teach the patients deep-breathing techniques. This triggers autonomic processes that are calming to the human body.

- Teach the patients visualization techniques, also called mental imagery. This involves visualizing a pleasant place or peaceful scene in their mind to induce a tranquil state (Valente, 1999).

- Urge the patients to meditate. Meditation is a technique to empty and cleanse the mind of all ego-based worries (Seaward, 2006; Townsend, 2015). Meditation emphasizes breathing and inner peace, focuses on concepts of comfort and emotional healing, relieves tension and anxiety, and promotes calm.

> ☑ **NOTE** Chapter 6, "Stress-Management Techniques," covers relaxation techniques like deep breathing, mental imagery, and meditation in more detail.

- Play music for the patients. If possible, do it in a room with good acoustics and a comfortable place to sit or lie down. Choose music with a slow tempo and no words (Seaward, 2006).

- Administer any sedating medications ordered, assess them for effectiveness, and monitor the patients for adverse effects.

After patients calm down and regain self-control, debrief with them to identify precipitating causes (Shelton, 1993). Educate them to recognize signs of escalating anxiety, and teach them to implement de-escalation interventions on their own to prevent future panic attacks.

The primary goals of treatment for anxiety and panic disorder are to reduce the severity of the symptoms and to prevent and treat any underlying medical conditions. By addressing these issues, patients can regain a sense of safety, self-control, and balance to their lives.

Test Yourself

PANIC DISORDER Darcy is a 28-year-old woman with a history of panic disorder. Today she has come to the hospital to visit her aunt, an inpatient who suffers from asthma. Darcy is accompanied by her daughter. Darcy appears alert, calm, and well-dressed.

When Darcy arrives, she walks up to the nurses station and politely asks for directions to her aunt's room. Darcy then proceeds to walk briskly down the hall to her aunt's room.

Fifteen minutes later, Darcy's aunt turns on her call light. She asks the responding nurse to come in and check on her visiting niece, who is "going wild." The nurse enters the room and sees Darcy pacing and pulling her hair out. Darcy has tears running down her cheeks. She yells loudly at the nurse, "I am going to catch asthma from her!" Darcy sits down and begins trembling and shaking. The nurse observes that Darcy is sweating profusely. Darcy yells, "I can't stand this! I am going to die!"

How would you handle this situation?

COMPARING CONDITIONS

Table 11.5 provides a comparison of schizophrenia, bipolar disorder, major depressive disorder, and panic disorder, including descriptions for each, assessment parameters, and suggested de-escalation techniques.

TABLE 11.5 A Comparison of Schizophrenia, Bipolar Disorder, Major Depressive Disorder, and Panic Disorder

Disorder Description	Assessment Parameters	De-Escalation Techniques
Schizophrenia		
Serious and lifelong mental disorder characterized by striking disturbances in mental functioning such as hallucinations, delusions, disorganized thinking, and lack of social engagement	Auditory or visual hallucinations Delusions Disorientation to reality Altered mental states Suicidal and/or homicidal ideation Agitated or aggressive behavior	Identify yourself to the patient. Speak slowly, clearly, and gently. Get help from a staff member who has established a rapport. Avoid laughing, joking, and whispering. Be honest. Keep promises. Encourage verbalization. Maintain an assertive yet friendly approach

continues

TABLE 11.5 **A Comparison of Schizophrenia, Bipolar Disorder, Major Depressive Disorder, and Panic Disorder** *(continued)*

Disorder Description	Assessment Parameters	De-Escalation Techniques
Schizophrenia *(continued)*		
		Provide a quiet environment with dim lights and no crowd.
		Engage in frequent observation of the patient (with one-to-one monitoring for patients who are suicidal or homicidal).
		Remove harmful or hazardous objects from environment.
		Redirect agitated behavior with physical activity.
		Ensure the staff conveys a calm attitude.
		Reorient the patient to reality.
Bipolar Disorder		
Mood disorder that manifests in cycles of intense mood swings that alternate between a manic state (characterized by exhilarated euphoria) and depressed states (marked by intense depression). In between are periods of normal mood and behavior. Bipolar disorder affects 2.6% of the U.S. adult population.	Mood swings Manic phase symptoms (refer to Table 11.1) Depressive phase symptoms (refer to Table 11.2)	Provide hydration, nutrition, and rest. Engage in frequent observation of the patient. Monitor for signs of suicidal ideation and complete a suicide risk assessment if indicated. Involve the patient in activities that require gross motor movements. Monitor medication effects, levels, and side effects. Encourage a short daytime nap. Assist with personal hygiene. Encourage self-care. Encourage diversional activities. Provide a quiet environment with dim lights and no crowd. Provide emotional support. Set realistic goals for behavior. Remove harmful or hazardous objects from environment. Set limits based in respect. Listen attentively. Avoid power struggles. Use a team approach. Teach relaxation techniques. Encourage verbalization.

Disorder Description	Assessment Parameters	De-Escalation Techniques
Major Depressive Disorder		
Disorder that is defined by the presence of five prominent depressive symptoms over a two-week period. (Refer to Table 11.3.) Symptoms cause substantial distress.	Depressive symptoms (refer to Table 11.3) History of suicide attempts Presence of suicidal thoughts, plan, intent, and means History of alcohol or drug abuse Isolation or withdrawal from family, friends, and/or community Disorientation or disorganization Anxiety Lifestyle Protective factors	Encourage verbalization. Encourage spirituality—for example, reading the Bible or another spiritual text. Encourage patient to read a book or magazine or watch TV. Encourage socialization. Teach problem-solving skills. Initiate suicide prevention plan. Teach positive coping skills for stress management. Develop therapeutic rapport. Provide constant observation for the actively suicidal. Teach relaxation techniques such as diaphragmic breathing, music, meditation, or yoga.
Panic Disorder		
A type of anxiety disorder characterized by a sudden episode of intense fear and anxiety. The episode develops suddenly for no apparent reason or precipitating event and triggers severe emotional reactions such as intense fear, apprehension, and feelings of doom.	Symptoms of panic attacks (refer to Table 11.4) Occurrence of anxiety Symptom duration and intensity Stressors and ongoing conflicts History of panic attacks Triggers of anxiety attacks	Remain with panicking patient. Provide reassurances of safety. Give emotional support. Use a slow, calm, and serene approach. Model calm. Speak in a brief, clear, and direct manner. Avoid touching the patient. Present reality to the patient. Provide directions one at a time. Provide a quiet environment with dim lights and no crowd. Allow the patient to pace. Encourage physical exercise. Encourage verbalization. Teach relaxation techniques such as deep breathing, mental imagery, music, and meditation. Monitor for medication side effects and adverse effects.

REFERENCES

Agency for Healthcare Research and Quality. (2007). *Roadmap to seclusion and restraint free mental health services.* Retrieved from https://innovations.ahrq.gov/qualitytools/roadmap-seclusion-and-restraint-free-mental-health-services

American Psychiatric Association. (2013). *Diagnostic and statistical manual of mental disorders (DSM-5).* Washington, DC: American Psychiatric Association.

Ballenger, J. C., & Fyer, A. J. (1993). Examining criteria for panic disorder. *Hospital and Community Psychiatry, 44*(3), 226–228.

Boyd, M. A. (2008). *Psychiatric nursing: Contemporary practice* (4th ed.). Philadelphia, PA: Lippincott, Williams & Wilkins.

Chabora, N., Judge-Gorny, M., & Grogan, K. (2003). The Four S Model in Action for de-escalation: An innovative state hospital-university collaborative endeavor. *Journal of Psychosocial Nursing and Mental Health Services, 41*(1), 22–28.

Copeland, D., & Henry, M. (2017). Workplace violence and perceptions of safety among emergency department staff members: Experiences, expectations, tolerance, reporting, and recommendations. *Journal of Trauma Nursing, 24*(2), 65–77. doi: 10.1097/JTN.0000000000000269

Edlund, M. J., & Swann, A. C. (1987). The economic and social costs of panic disorder. *Hospital and Community Psychiatry, 38*(12), 1,277–1,288.

Gagné, G. G., Furman, M. J., Carpenter, L. L., & Price, L. H. (2000). Efficacy of continuation ECT and antidepressant drugs compared to long-term antidepressants alone in depressed patients. *The American Journal of Psychiatry, 157*(12), 1,960–1,965.

Gately, L. A., & Stabb, S. D., (2005). Psychology students' training in the management of potentially violent clients. *Professional Psychology: Research and Practice, 36*(6), 681–687.

Goldberg. R. J. (1998). *Practical guide to the care of the psychiatric patient* (2nd ed.). St. Louis, MO: Mosby.

Harris, E. C., & Barraclough, B. (1999). Suicide as an outcome for mental disorders: A meta-analysis. *The British Journal of Psychiatry, 170,* 205–208.

Hilgers, J. (2003). Comforting a confused patient. *Nursing, 33*(1), 48–50.

Hodgins, S. (2008). Violent behaviour among people with schizophrenia: A framework for investigations of causes, and effective treatment, and prevention. *Philosophical Transactions of the Royal Society of London, Series B, Biological Sciences, 363*(1503), 2,505–2,518. doi: 10.1098/rstb.2008.0034

Jeffrey, D., & Austen, S. (2005). Adapting de-escalation techniques with deaf service users. *Nursing Standard, 19*(49), 41–47.

Kane, J. M. (2003). Review of treatments that can ameliorate nonadherence in patients with schizophrenia. *The Journal of Clinical Psychology, 67*(Suppl 5), 9–14.

Karasu, B., Gelenberg, A., Wang, P., & Merriam, A. (2000). Practice guidelines for the treatment of patients with major depression disorder (Revision). *American Journal of Psychiatry, 157*(4 Suppl), 1–45.

Lehman, A. F., Lieberman, J. A., Dixon, L. B., McGlashan, T. H., Miller, A. L., Perkins, D. O., ... American Psychiatric Association Steering Committee on Practice Guidelines. (2004). Practice guideline for the treatment of patients with schizophrenia (2nd ed.). *The American Journal of Psychiatry, 161*(2 Suppl), 1–56.

McGrandles, A., & McCaig, M. (2013). Diagnosis and management of anxiety in primary care. *Nurse Prescribing, 8*(7), 310–318.

Minzenberg, M. J., Yoon, J. H., & Carter, C. S. (2011). Schizophrenia. In R. E. Hales, S. C. Yudofsky, & G. O. Gabbard (Eds.), *The American Psychiatric Publishing textbook of clinical psychiatry* (5th ed.), pp. 1–36. St. Louis, MO: American Psychiatric Publishing, Inc.

Pollard, C. A., Obermeier, H. J., & Cox, G. L. (1987). Inpatient treatment of complicated agoraphobia and panic disorder. *Hospital and Community Psychiatry, 38*(9), 951–958.

Sargent, M. (1990). Panic disorder. *Hospital and Community Psychiatry, 41*(6), 621–623.

Seaward, B. L. (2012). *Managing stress: Principles and strategies for health and well-being* (7th ed.). Burlington, VT: Jones & Bartlett Learning.

Shelton, R. C. (1993). Pharmacology of panic disorder. *Hospital and Community Psychiatry, 44*(8), 725–726.

Tompkins, O. (2010). Panic attacks. *AAOHN, 58*(6), 268–269.

Townsend, M. C. (2015). *Psychiatric mental health nursing: Concepts of care in evidence-based practice* (8th ed.). Philadelphia, PA: F. A. Davis Company.

Valente, S. M. (1999). Anxiety and panic disorders in older adults. *Home Health Care Management & Practice, 11*(4), 49–59.

DE-ESCALATION OF PATIENTS EXHIBITING NON-SUICIDAL SELF-INJURY (NSSI) BEHAVIOR

"When you make peace with yourself, you make peace with the world."

–Maha Ghosananda

OBJECTIVES

- Examine origins of NSSI behavior

- Explore how to assess patients with NSSI behavior

- Find out how to prevent escalation of patients with NSSI behavior

- Define de-escalation practices for patients with NSSI behavior

- Explore differences between patients with NSSI behavior and patients with suicidal ideation

Non-suicidal self-injury (NSSI) behavior is defined as deliberate behavior that results in a self-inflicted injury and the destruction of body tissue *without* a conscious suicidal intent. NSSI involves deliberately mutilating the body—for example, by cutting or burning. Individuals who engage in NSSI repeatedly inflict shallow yet painful injuries to their body and skin. NSSI behavior causes significant distress and often interferes in academic, interpersonal, and other important areas of normal life.

> ☑ **NOTE** NSSI behavior was previously described as self-mutilation, self-inflicted violence, self-injurious behavior, or self-directed violence (Agüero, Medina, Obradovich, & Berner, 2018).

The *DSM-5* identifies the criteria for NSSI in its section for conditions requiring further study. It describes NSSI behavior as five or more days of intentional self-inflicted injury to one's body likely to cause bleeding, bruising, or pain (American Psychiatric Association [APA], 2013). Individuals who engage in NSSI express no suicidal intent. They are aware the behavior will not result in death. The *DSM-5* further defines NSSI behavior as being conducted to obtain relief from negative feelings such as depression, anxiety, or distress; to resolve an interpersonal difficulty; or to induce positive feelings. Table 12.1 lists types of behaviors associated with NSSI.

TABLE 12.1 Behaviors Associated With NSSI

Cutting	Scratching
Cigarette burns	Self-embedding objects
Scalding	Ingesting objects
Biting self	Skin picking
Hair pulling	Stabbing self
Head banging	Ingesting toxins
Striking self	Excessive rubbing with evisceration of tissue

NSSI is usually inflicted with a knife, needle, razor, or other sharp instrument. For example, someone who engages in NSSI might use a razor to cut or scratch their skin or embed a sharp object such as a sewing needle under the skin. Injuries are generally superficial but may deepen with repetition. NSSI can begin with relatively benign practices such as hair-pulling but escalate—for example, to intentional self-burning, scalding, or biting (Mental Health Foundation & Camelot Foundation, 2006) or to the ingestion of objects or toxic substances. This can lead to accidental suicide. Employing multiple methods of injury is associated with more severe psychopathology, including suicide attempts (APA, 2013).

> ☑ **NOTE** At least 80% of NSSI behavior involves stabbing or cutting the skin with a sharp object (Greydanus & Shek, 2009; Hawton, Zahl, & Weatherall, 2003; Idig-Camuroglu & Gölge, 2018).

NSSI should be distinguished from behaviors such as tattooing or body piercing. In other words, NSSI is the deliberate, non–life threatening, self-inflicted bodily injury or disfigurement of a socially unacceptable nature (APA, 2013). NSSI is also different from behaviors that may occur during psychotic episodes, delirium, or substance use or withdrawal or that are related to any other mental or medical disorder.

The most common self-injurers are adolescents with no history of mental health issues. Adolescents with a history of neglect or abuse or who are victims of bullying (including cyber-bullying) are at a higher risk for NSSI. Adults with a history of psychological trauma are also more susceptible to NSSI (van der Kolk, 1989a), as are adults with psychosis and auditory hallucinations.

> ☑ **NOTE** Statistics show that as many as 4% of American adults self-injure, with more than 1% of the general population engaging in chronic or severe self-injury. Between 24% and 40% of mental health patients self-injure. NSSI typically begins in the early teen years, with inpatient hospitalization peaking between ages 20 and 29 (APA, 2013; Kerr, Muehlenkamp, & Turner, 2010; Williams & Bydalek, 2007).

ORIGINS OF NSSI BEHAVIOR

There is no single origin of NSSI behavior. Every individual self-injures for a different reason. However, self-injury is almost always used as a coping mechanism when individuals no longer feel they are able to resolve their issues using standard problem-solving techniques (Alderman, 1997; Hawton et al., 2003; Klonsky, 2007).

Some people self-injure to relieve or distract from emotional pain. Self-injurers often report an immediate sense of relief from intense or overwhelming negative emotions—such as tension, anxiety, depression, stress, emotional numbness, feelings of failure, and self-hatred—when they engage in the injurious behavior. Other people self-injure as a form of self-punishment, which they believe they deserve, or as an expression of self-hate (APA, 2013).

> ☑ **NOTE** When an individual self-injures, such as by cutting himself, the person's body releases endorphins to reduce the pain. These endorphins may soothe and calm the person.

Here are other common reasons for NSSI behavior:

- **Relief from dissociation.** Individuals who feel physically or emotionally detached from their body due to past emotional traumas may cut themselves just to feel *something*—even if it's pain. Similarly, individuals might self-injure simply to feel they are alive.

- **To communicate emotional pain.** For some, self-injury is an attempt to communicate pain that cannot be expressed in spoken words.

- **Peer pressure.** Adolescents sometimes self-injure in groups as a result of peer pressure. In some cases, this "group" might consist of visitors to a website devoted to self-injury.

- **In response to environmental triggers.** Most self-injurious behavior is in response to interpersonal conflicts in the home environment. Self-invalidation that triggers self-injury is learned from environments in which being punished, disregarded, criticized, or trivialized is common.

- **To manipulate others.** For some people who self-injure, it's an attempt to manipulate or control others (APA, 2013; Dear, Thompson, Howells, & Hall, 2001).

NSSI, Borderline Personality Disorder, and Other Disorders

NSSI behavior is a primary symptom of borderline personality disorder. Often, people who suffer from this disorder engage in NSSI behavior in an attempt to manipulate or control others. NSSI behavior is also associated with eating disorders, substance use disorders, post-traumatic stress disorder, schizophrenia, anxiety, and depressive disorders (Fox & Hawton, 2004).

Learning theory may provide another rationale for NSSI behavior:

> According to learning theory, a child or adolescent may engage in self-injurious behavior, such as stereotyped head banging or impulsive skin cutting, either to gain access to something that they experience as pleasant, such as social attention, which is contingent on performance of the self-injurious act (positive reinforcement), or to escape from something that they experience as unpleasant, such as social demands, suspension of which is contingent on performance of the self-injurious act (negative reinforcement). (Barrett, 2008, p. 872)

In both cases, says Barrett, "when self-injury results in access to a pleasant condition or facilitates escape from an unpleasant circumstance, the result is a strengthening (reinforcement) of the self-injurious behavior" (2008, p. 872).

Another explanation pertains to object constancy. Some individuals who exhibit NSSI behavior cannot tolerate conflict, which they equate with the total loss of the relationship. In other words, they have an inability to formulate object constancy (Hicks & Hinck, 2008). The feelings of abandonment that inevitably ensue—even when only imagined—may cause severe anxiety that results in NSSI behavior.

> **⚠ CAUTION** Regardless of the specific reason a person self-injures, the behavior can sometimes become addictive. When this happens, the individual craves the release of self-injury.

ASSESSING PATIENTS WITH NSSI BEHAVIOR

When assessing a patient who exhibits NSSI behavior, ask some variation on the following questions:

- **When or in what circumstances does the behavior typically occur?** This can help you identify potential causes or triggers for the behavior (Townsend, 2015). With this information in hand, you can ensure the person is not exposed to these triggers until there is emotional stability.

- **What type of self-injury do you most commonly inflict?** Examples might include cutting or burning.

- **On what area of the body is injury most commonly inflicted?** Examples might be on the arm, legs, or face.

- **What instrument is most commonly used to self-injure?** Examples could include a knife, glass, or a sharp piece of metal.

- **What coping skills do you use to keep the urges to self-harm under control?** Examples could include reading a book, going for a walk, or talking to a friend. If these interventions have worked in the past to prevent self-injury, they will most likely also be effective in the future to prevent harm.

These are vital questions to ask to prevent self-injury. When these questions are answered, the nurse will know where to observe for self-injury and what types of harming instrument to prevent access to for safety. The nurse should enter the patient's answers to these questions in the treatment plan to prevent future self-injury.

> ✅ **NOTE**   When assessing the patient, try to determine whether the NSSI behavior occurs in response to increasing anxiety, and what is triggering that anxiety, to ascertain how to prevent future self-injury.

PREVENTING ESCALATION OF PATIENTS WITH NSSI BEHAVIOR

The following interventions can help you prevent patients who exhibit NSSI behavior from escalating (in other words, engaging in those behaviors). Your primary goal here is to teach the patient positive coping skills to manage stress in a healthy manner.

- **Observe the patient's behavior.** Patients who engage in NSSI need more frequent monitoring to protect them from self-injury. Some at-risk patients might even require one-to-one observation.

- **Ask the patient to report urges to self-injure.** This gives you an opportunity to prevent the self-injury.

- **Encourage the patient to verbalize.** Discussing feelings with a trusted staff member (like you) can provide a degree of relief and may help prevent self-injury. This is especially true if you convey an attitude of acceptance and view the patient as a worthwhile individual.

- **Encourage the patient to engage in physical exercise.** Physical outlets like isometric exercise, jogging, or a long walk can help defuse the pent-up tension and anxiety that can lead to self-injury.

- **Try the "rubber band" trick.** Ask the patient to wear a loose rubber band around the wrist and to snap it (rather than cutting, for example) when there's an urge to self-harm.

- **Use ice.** Having the patient hold an ice cube or rub it on his or her body until it melts can help relieve urges to self-harm.

- **Use a red marker.** Having the patient draw on his or her skin with a red water-soluble felt-tip pen (rather than cutting, for example) may be beneficial (Boyd, 2008; Dresser, 1999; Klonsky & Glenn, 2008; Mental Health Foundation & Camelot Foundation, 2006).

- **Encourage the patient to write in a journal.** Writing about their feelings and experiences can provide patients with emotional relief. Patients can also write a list of their negative feelings and then tear it up to relieve stress.

- **Encourage the patient to create.** Making artwork such as collages can help relieve the patient's urge to self-injure.

- **Turn on some music.** Music with a slow tempo and no words can help calm patients down and prevent self-injury.

- **Be a role model.** Show the patient what appropriate behavior looks like.

- **Give praise.** When the patient resists the urge to self-harm, offer positive reinforcement such as a smile or a kind word.

DE-ESCALATION TECHNIQUES FOR PATIENTS WITH NSSI BEHAVIOR

If a patient self-injures while in your care, it's critical that you care for the wounds in a matter-of-fact manner. Do not offer sympathy or additional attention. This will simply reinforce the patient's behavior. Refusing to give undue attention to this maladaptive behavior may help prevent the patient from repeating it in the future. Do, however, encourage the patient to verbalize any feelings experienced before engaging in the behavior. Helping the patient become aware of precipitating factors can help resolve the triggering issues and prevent reoccurrence (Townsend, 2015).

Reversing NSSI

Fortunately, NSSI is reversible if recognized early and treated. Therapy for NSSI is very beneficial, especially if the individual is motivated to change and recover (Armstrong, Owen, Roberts, & Koch, 2002). Available therapies for NSSI include the following:

- **Cognitive behavioral therapy (CBT).** This helps patients establish healthy ways of successfully managing stress—*without* NSSI. An example of a CBT technique is mindfulness meditation to relieve stress and convey self-acceptance.

- **Dialectical behavioral therapy (DBT).** This is one of the best therapies for positive, long-term improvement in the prevention of NSSI (Suyemoto, 1998). DBT uses behavioral and cognitive strategies to prevent self-injury. The focus of this therapy is to directly suppress urges to self-harm or to eliminate access to self-harming means.

In addition, the depressive symptoms that often underlie NSSI can be treated with prescribed antidepressant medication.

TEST YOURSELF

NSSI BEHAVIOR Judy is a 26-year-old, alert, well-dressed woman admitted to a medical healthcare facility for a respiratory infection. During the admission assessment, Judy admits to self-injury during times of stress. Judy has scars and small cut marks on both legs. She also has a recent cigarette burn on her left wrist. When questioned about the wounds, Judy explains, "I had an argument with my mother" and "I cut to feel better." Judy goes on to say, "I saw my mother yesterday. That's when I burned my wrist." Finally, Judy says, "My mother doesn't want me to drink with my friends" and "I have to burn my wrist sometimes, but it's better afterwards."

How would you handle this situation?

DIFFERENTIATING NSSI BEHAVIOR FROM SUICIDAL IDEATION

There are substantial differences between NSSI and suicidal ideation. Table 12.2 outlines these differences.

TABLE 12.2 **Differences Between NSSI and Suicidal Ideation**

NSSI	Suicidal Ideation
Patients who engage in NSSI do not have a specific intention to kill themselves.	Suicidal behaviors reflect a deliberate intention to end life.
NSSI involves nonlethal means and results only in superficial damage to the person's body.	Suicide involves highly lethal means and can result in serious physical damage or death.
The goal of NSSI is to cope with stressors to feel better.	The goal of suicide is to feel nothing at all.
Individuals engage in NSSI as a way to sustain life.	Suicide is meant to end life.
After NSSI, patients experience decreased distress and an improved emotional state (Brausch & Gutierrez, 2010). They feel better.	For individuals engaged in suicidal ideation, emotional pain is seen as unending and unbearable suffering. After surviving a suicide attempt, the person feels much worse even than before the attempt and emotionally spent by the physical stressors associated with surviving.

> ☑ **NOTE** Research indicates patients who self-injure have fewer depressed symptoms, less suicidal ideation, greater self-esteem, and greater parental support than suicidal patients (Brausch & Gutierrez, 2010).

That being said, NSSI is a strong risk indicator for future suicide (Low, Jones, MacLeod, Power, & Duggan, 2002; van der Kolk, 1989b). Indeed, research shows that individuals who self-harm have an increased risk of suicide in the long term. This is especially true for adolescent males (Arsenault-Lapierre, Kim, & Turecki, 2004; Hawton et al., 2016). In 40% to 60% of suicides, there is evidence of self-injury occurring within the previous one-year period. Research indicates that adolescents who self-injure have double the risk of the general population of dying by suicide (Resch, Parzer, Brunner, & BELLA study group, 2008). Fortunately, with early detection and intervention and effective treatment, there is great hope for recovery for patients who engage in NSSI or suicidal ideation.

REFERENCES

Agüero, G., Medina, V., Obradovich, G., & Berner, E. (2018). Self-injurious behaviors among adolescents. A qualitative study of characteristics, meanings, and contexts. *Archivos Argentinos de Pediatría*, *116*(6), 394–401.

Alderman, T. (1997). *The scarred soul: Understanding and ending self-inflicted violence*. Oakland, CA: New Harbinger Publications.

American Psychiatric Association. (2013). *Diagnostic and statistical manual of mental disorders (DSM-5)*. Washington, DC: American Psychiatric Association.

Armstrong, M. L., Owen, D. C., Roberts, A. E., & Koch, J. R. (2002). College students and tattoos: Influence of image, identity, family, and friends. *Journal of Psychosocial Nursing and Mental Health Services, 40*(10), 20–29.

Arsenault-Lapierre, G, Kim, C., & Turecki, G. (2004). Psychiatric diagnoses in 3275 suicides: A meta-analysis. *BMC Psychiatry, 4*, 37.

Barrett, R. P. (2008). Atypical behavior: Self-injury and pica. In M. L. Wolraich, P. H. Dworkin, D. D. Drotar, & E. C. Perrin (Eds.), *Developmental-behavioral pediatrics: evidence and practice*, pp. 871–885. Philadelphia, PA: Mosby.

Boyd, M. A. (2008). *Psychiatric nursing: Contemporary practice* (4th ed.). Philadelphia, PA: Lippincott, Williams & Wilkins.

Brausch, A. M., & Gutierrez, P. M. (2010). Differences in non-suicidal self-injury and suicide attempts in adolescents. *Journal of Youth and Adolescence, 39*(3), 233–242.

Dear, G. E., Thompson, D. M., Howells, K., & Hall, G. J. (2001). Self-harm in Western Australian prisons: Differences between prisoners who have self-harmed and those who have not. *Australian and New Zealand Journal of Criminology, 34*(3), 277–292.

Dresser, J. G. (1999). Wrapping: A technique for interrupting self-mutilation. *Journal of the American Psychiatric Nurses Association, 5*(2), 67–70.

Fox, C., & Hawton, K. (2004). *Deliberate self-harm in adolescence*. London, UK: Jessica Kingsley Publishers.

Greydanus, D. E., & Shek, D. (2009). Deliberate self-harm and suicide in adolescents. *The Keio Journal of Medicine, 58*(3), 144–151.

Hawton, K., Witt, K. G., Salisbury, T. L. T., Arensman, E., Gunnell, D., Hazell, P., … van Heeringen, K. (2016). Psychosocial interventions following self-harm in adults: A systemic review and meta-analysis. *The Lancet, 3*(8), 740–750. doi: 10.1016/S2215-0366(16)30070-0

Hawton, K., Zahl, D., & Weatherall, R. (2003). Suicide following deliberate self-harm: Long-term follow-up of patients who presented to a general hospital. *The British Journal of Psychiatry, 182*, 537–542.

Hicks, K. M., & Hinck, S. M. (2008). Concept analysis of self-mutilation. *Journal of Advanced Nursing, 64*(4), 408–413.

Idig-Camuroglu, M., & Gölge, Z. B. (2018). Non-suicidal self-injury among university students in Turkey: The effect of gender and childhood abuse. *Psychiatria Danubina, 30*(4), 410–420.

Kerr, P. L., Muehlenkamp, J. J., & Turner, J. M. (2010). Nonsuicidal self-injury: A review of current research for family and primary care physicians. *Journal of American Board of Family Medicine, 23*(2), 240–259. doi: 10.3122/jabfm.2010.02.090110

Klonsky, E. D. (2007). The functions of deliberate self-injury: A review of the evidence. *Clinical Psychology Review, 27*(2), 226–239.

Klonsky, E. D., & Glenn, C. R. (2008). Resisting urges to self-injure. *Behavioral and Cognitive Psychotherapy, 36*(2), 211–220. doi: 10.1017/S1352465808004128

Low, G., Jones, D., MacLeod, A., Power, M., & Duggan, C. (2002). Childhood trauma, dissociation and self-harming behavior: A pilot study. *The British Journal of Medical Psychology, 73*, 269–278.

Mental Health Foundation & Camelot Foundation. (2006). The truth hurts: Report of the national inquiry into self-harm among young people. *Mental Health Foundation*. Retrieved from https://www.mentalhealth.org.uk/publications/truth-hurts-report1

Resch, F., Parzer, P., Brunner, R., & BELLA study group. (2008). Self-mutilation and suicidal behavior in children and adolescents: Prevalence and psychosocial correlates: Results of the BELLA study. *European Child & Adolescent Psychiatry, 17*(Suppl 1), 92–98. doi: 10.1007/s00787-008-1010-3

Suyemoto, K. L. (1998). The functions of self-mutilation. *Clinical Psychology Review, 18*(5), 531–554.

Townsend, M. C. (2015). *Psychiatric mental health nursing: Concepts of care in evidence-based practice* (8th ed.). Philadelphia, PA: F. A. Davis Company.

van der Kolk, B. A. (1989a). The compulsion to repeat the trauma: Re-enactment, revictimization, and masochism. *The Psychiatric Clinics of North America, 12*(2), 389–411.

van der Kolk, B. A. (1989b). *Psychological trauma*. Washington, DC: American Psychiatric Press.

Williams, K. A., & Bydalek, K. A. (2007). Adolescent self-mutilation: Diagnosis & treatment. *Journal of Psychosocial Nursing and Mental Health Services, 45*(12), 19–23.

DE-ESCALATION OF PATIENTS WITH DEMENTIA

"Every soul is beautiful and precious; is worthy of dignity and respect, and deserving of peace, joy and love."

–Bryan H. McGill

OBJECTIVES

- Study assessment criteria for dementia

- Find out how to prevent dementia patients from escalating

- Identify effective de-escalation techniques for dementia patients

- Consider the importance of maintaining quality of life for dementia patients

Dementia is a syndrome characterized by generalized progressive cognitive deterioration impairing both social and vocational functioning. Dementia results in changes of behavior, perception, memory, problem-solving abilities, and judgment that interfere with normal daily life and functions (American Psychiatric Association [APA], 2013; Kneisl & Trigoboff, 2009).

The *DSM-5* lists dementia under a new name: major neurocognitive disorder. It describes diagnostic criteria as a significant cognitive decline from a previous level of performance in one or more cognitive domains. These cognitive domains include complex attention, executive function, learning and memory, language, perceptual-motor, and social cognition. (It should be noted that the cognitive deficits do not occur exclusively in the context of delirium [APA, 2013].) Concerns about cognitive deficits might be expressed by the individual, a knowledgeable informant, or a clinician. Declines in cognitive performance are ideally documented by standardized neuropsychological testing or another quantified clinical assessment.

A prominent type of dementia is neurocognitive disorder due to Alzheimer's disease. Neurocognitive disorders of the Alzheimer's variety have multiple possible causes, including acetylcholine alterations, plaque, and tangles in the brain. In addition, there is a possible genetic predisposition to Alzheimer's disease. Head trauma may also be a factor in development of Alzheimer's.

Dementia interferes with the individual's ability to maintain independence and to perform everyday tasks. At a minimum, patients who suffer from dementia will require assistance with complex instrumental activities of daily living such as paying bills and managing medications.

> ✅ **NOTE** Between 1.4% and 1.6% of Americans between the ages of 65 and 69 suffer from dementia; the percentages climb to 16% to 25% for those over age 85. Nearly 5.2 million Americans over 65 have dementia. Dementia is the fourth most prevalent cause of death in adult populations (APA, 2013; Townsend, 2015).

ASSESSING A DEMENTIA PATIENT

Nurses must be aware of early warning signs of dementia. Examples of early warning signs are if a person:

- Repeatedly asks the same question or repeats the same answer over and over

- Has trouble organizing time, such as a work or social schedule

- Forgets to pay bills on time

- Frequently misplaces objects

- Forgets to bathe or has poor personal hygiene (e.g., has body odor, dirt under fingernails, tangled hair, or mussed clothing) (Kneisl & Trigoboff, 2009; Schuurmans, Duursma, & Shortridge-Baggett, 2001)

- Wears clothing that is inappropriate for the season

- Demonstrates apathy in affect (facial expression) and demeanor

- Has trouble learning or remembering new information

- Forgets the names of family members

- Forgets to take regularly scheduled medications

- Frequently misses scheduled medical appointments

- Loses the ability to add and subtract basic numbers (APA, 2013; National Institute for Health and Clinical Excellence [NICE], 2006; Schuurmans et al., 2001)

- Finds it difficult to remember recent conversations or events

Other early signs of dementia include anxiety, depression, frustration, agitation, and a heightened sense of suspicion (Woods, Rapp, & Beck, 2004).

Dementia signs and symptoms in the mid to late stages of the disease are very prevalent. Examples of mid- to late-stage signs and symptoms are if a person:

- Exhibits poor awareness of safety such as walking into oncoming traffic

- Wears inappropriate layers of clothing, such as a heavy coat in summer

- Forgets to completely dress before going out in public

- Gets lost in familiar areas (APA, 2013; NICE, 2006; Schuurmans et al., 2001)

- Experiences disturbances in sleep/wake patterns, such as sleeping all day and then staying up all night

- Experiences weight loss due to appetite changes or simply forgetting to eat

- Exhibits an inability to perform motor tasks

- Exhibits diminished hand-eye coordination and gait

■ Is unable to select the correct word or uses a wrong word when speaking

■ Shows persistent disorientation with regard to person, time, and place (APA, 2013; Schuurmans et al., 2001)

■ Experiences uncontrolled urinary and fecal incontinence.

TEST YOURSELF

DEMENTIA George Watson is a 92-year-old man admitted to a healthcare facility with a diagnosis of dementia. Mr. Watson has been living with his daughter for several years. He had surgery four days ago for an open reduction of a fractured clavicle and has remained in the hospital for observation since then.

Mr. Watson is increasingly forgetful, confused, and suspicious, as well as gruff in his interactions with staff. He has begun wandering into other patients' rooms and becomes agitated and aggressive when he is redirected to his correct room. Mr. Watson shakes his fist and shouts loudly at staff members, "I am in my right room! All of you just leave!"

How would you handle this situation?

PREVENTING ESCALATION WITH DEMENTIA PATIENTS

As always, it's better to prevent a patient from escalating to an agitated or aggressive state than to try to de-escalate the patient after the fact. There are several steps you can take to prevent dementia patients from escalating.

One effective practice is to retain a consistent and stable healthcare staff. That way the caregiver will be familiar to the dementia patient. Put procedures in place for handling dementia patients during shift changes, such as introducing patients to the nurses on the next shift, for a smooth changeover (Keane, 2006). Also avoid switching the patient to a different room or moving furniture around in the patient's room (NICE, 2006; Power, 2010). Maintain a comforting and familiar environment. Keep the patient's room well lit so there's a clear view of surroundings, and keep noise levels down to prevent the patient from becoming overwhelmed. Finally, elevate the head of the patient's bed for comfort and safety. Providing comfort measures such as these improves the patient's disposition and reduces the risk of escalation.

Another helpful measure is to provide clear explanations of all medical procedures. When assisting a patient with a procedure, explain each step along the way, as well as possible outcomes. This helps to reduce fear that may trigger agitation (Hoe, Jesnick, Turner, Leavey, & Livingston, 2017). On a related note, the skill and efficiency with which the procedures is carried out also has an effect. In other words, if you perform the procedure skillfully and efficiently, the patient is less likely to become agitated or aggressive.

When communicating with the patient about medical procedures—or anything else—keep these points in mind:

- Take a calm, caring approach (Huis In Het Veld et al., 2016). In this way you can help keep the patient calm while also serving as a role model.

- Spend time talking with the patient and actively listen to develop therapeutic rapport. Active positive listening also helps to de-escalate agitated patients.

- When the patient has a problem, allow verbalization about it, and validate the concerns (Ledgerd et al., 2016).

- Be respectful and polite. Use honorifics like "sir" and "ma'am," and employ simple courtesies like saying "please" and "thank you."

- Provide a schedule of daily activities and procedures. This will help the patient prepare for the day.

- Hang seasonal decorations. This will help the patient remember the time of year.

- Display photos of loved ones in the patient's room (Boyle, 2006; Kneisl & Trigoboff, 2009). This helps the patient remember who's who. (A photo album can serve the same purpose.)

- Bring in items from home. Ask a family member to bring items from home for placement in the patient's room. This will make the patient's surroundings feel more familiar.

- Display items related to the patient's hobbies or interests. These can serve as cues to jog the patient's memory.

- Be flexible. Accommodate the patient's fluctuating physical and mental abilities to help stave off frustration and anger.

Pet Therapy

Some nursing homes use pet therapy to comfort patients with dementia and to promote appropriate behavior. Pet therapy is a form of animal-assisted therapy that involves the purposeful use of animals to provide affection and attention to patients in long-term care facilities to help them to relax. Often dogs or cats are offered for pet therapy. These animals are trained to respond in a calm, nonthreatening manner to patients. Patients are allowed to stroke or pet the animals, providing the comfort of touch. Some facilities have enclosed aviaries for birds. Patients often enjoy watching the birds fly about and build nests and listening to the birds twitter and sing. Pet therapy is considered a beneficial form of diversional therapy for comfort and calming.

Guidelines for Dementia Care

The purpose of dementia care is to restore function and preserve quality of life. Here are some guidelines for caring for patients with dementia:

- **Encourage patients to practice self-care.** This fosters independence, builds self-esteem, and preserves physical abilities.

- **Establish simple routines.** This makes the routines easier to remember and helps preserve executive function.

- **Use visual cues.** For example, prominently display a photo outside the patients' doors to help them find their rooms.

- **Organize activities and opportunities to socialize.** These should be appropriate to the patients' cognitive levels.

- **Provide positive reinforcement.** When the patients exhibit appropriate behavior, offer a smile, a pat on the back, verbal praise, or a reward.

- **Promote physical exercise.** Encourage the patients to participate in physical activities that they enjoy, and allow them to go at their own pace.

- **Protect the patients' privacy and dignity.** When assisting the patients with bathing, use the minimum number of staff needed for the procedure, and close all doors, blinds, or drapes to provide personal privacy for dressing.

When caring for a patient with dementia, the focus is on safety and on reaching the highest possible levels of functioning (NICE, 2006; Varcarolis, 2011).

EFFECTIVE DE-ESCALATION PRACTICES FOR DEMENTIA PATIENTS

Effective de-escalation interventions for dementia patients encompass multiple domains of care. One effective intervention is verbal de-escalation—in other words, encouraging the patient to talk out any issues. For example, if a dementia patient shouts, "I feel so angry, I want to jump up and down and scream!" you might reply with, "Tell me about what happened that is upsetting you." This can help the patient ventilate the emotion and defuse hostility and anger.

Relaxation techniques such as deep breathing, meditation, and progressive muscular relaxation exercises are also calming to those with dementia (Agency for Healthcare Research and Quality (AHRQ), 2011; Power, 2010; Russell-Williams et al., 2018). Other relaxation techniques include the following:

- **Aromatherapy.** This involves diffusing a pleasant scent throughout the environment to soothe and calm.

- **Comfort measures.** For example, giving the patient a back massage can help in relaxation. The comfort of human touch is calming for dementia-related symptoms. (Remember: Always ask for permission before touching a patient in this way.)

- **Isometric exercise.** Isometric exercises are contractions of particular muscles or muscle groups to build strength. The calming motion of the simple exercises helps dementia patients relax.

- **Relaxation recordings.** Listening to relaxation recordings can be soothing and calming to those with dementia (Keane, 2006; Power, 2010).

Multisensory stimulation—the therapeutic use of music or dancing—is also soothing for dementia patients (Kales, Gitlin, Lyketsos, & Detroit Expert Panel on Assessment and Management of Neuropsychiatric Symptoms of Dementia, 2014).

If dementia patients appear angry, your first response should be to ask them if they are in pain (Husebo, Achterberg, & Flo, 2016). Individuals with dementia sometimes have difficulty clearly communicating physical issues to others; irritable or belligerent behavior might in fact be an indicator of physical pain (Husebo, Ballard, Cohen-Mansfield, Seifert, & Aarsland, 2014). In this case, de-escalation may be as easy as offering patients an acetaminophen pill.

> ☑ **NOTE** When dementia patients exhibit inappropriate behavior, it is rarely intentional. More often it is a result of a misunderstanding or simply frustration with their disabilities or discomfort. Or, they might not understand or remember what is expected.

If that doesn't work, there are other steps you can take to calm angry or agitated patients. One is to distract or redirect their attention. To begin, calmly and firmly tell them "no," and remind them of your expectations with regard to behavior (Bair, Toth, Johnson, Rosenberg, & Hurdle, 1999). Then redirect the patients' attention to a calming activity that they enjoy (Savage, Crawford, & Nashed, 2004). For example, you might encourage them to watch TV or distract them by giving them a stuffed animal to hold (Rueve & Welton, 2008). Engaging patients in this higher-level activity can help keep them interested, busy, and calm.

> ❓ **TIP** If dementia patients become agitated while attempting to complete a task, try simplifying the task. This increases the chances that they will be able to complete the task and can help to quell their frustration.

Reminiscence therapy is another technique for de-escalating agitated or angry dementia patients. As discussed in Chapter 4, "De-Escalation Techniques," this simply involves asking people to think about a pleasant event in the past, such as their wedding day or the birth of their first grandchild. This can help the patients calm down (Power, 2010).

Managing Patient Grief

Often, dementia patients will express a desire to see a loved one who is deceased. How you respond is key to helping the patient remain calm. For example, if 92-year-old dementia patient Jean says she wants to see her father, don't say, "No, you can't see your father. Your father is dead." If you do, the patient will likely experience the same grief she felt when her father died—even if it was decades before. This may cause her to cry for hours or fly into a rage. To prevent this, try saying, "Your father sounds like a wonderful person. Tell me about him!" As the patient begins to talk about her father, she will calm down and begin to remember the loss so many years ago in a kinder and gentler manner, without traumatic effects (Savage et al., 2004).

De-escalation techniques for confused (rather than angry) dementia patients are a bit different. Your goal here is to reorient the patient to reality and clear up any misconceptions. To start, when you approach the patient, introduce yourself (even if you've worked with the patient plenty of times before) and address the patient using a formal name. Then reassure the patient of safety and explain everything you are doing to help. When communicating with the patient, use short, simple phrases and maintain eye contact.

> **? TIP**   To help prevent dementia patients from becoming confused, provide clocks and calendars so they can keep track of the date and time (Varcarolis, 2011). Also encourage patients to wear prescribed glasses or hearing aids to reduce confusion and agitation.

CASE STUDY

DEMENTIA

Mr. Carson is a 75-year-old man with dementia who was admitted to a medical center for treatment of pancreatitis. Mr. Carson is forgetful but has been polite in interactions with nurses.

At 10 p.m., Mr. Carson turns on his call light and requests that the nurse come to "remove" someone from his room. When the nurse enters the darkened room, Mr. Carson points to a dark shadowy corner and says, "There is a strange man standing there. I am frightened. Tell him to leave." The nurse sees no one in the corner. She turns on the lights to fully illuminate the room so the patient can see properly. The nurse then calmly says to the patient, "See Mr. Carson, there is no one in the corner. It's just a shadow on a chair." This helps to clarify reality. The nurse continues, "Mr. Carson, you are safe here. I will be glad to sit with you for a while and we can talk." This helps to reassure Mr. Carson that he is safe.

MAINTAINING QUALITY OF LIFE FOR DEMENTIA PATIENTS

Best practices in dementia care are patient-centered and focused on mental health, wellness, and recovery. There is real potential to promote well-being in individuals with dementia (AHRQ, 2011). Despite significant losses, these patients can continue to find joy and fulfillment in life. Nurses must offer hope and dispel fears for those with dementia.

Nurses must do the same for the dementia patient's family, friends, and other caregivers—in addition to encouraging them to take on a supportive role in the patient's care and to explore resources to improve the patient's quality of life (as well as their own). Fostering an atmosphere of inclusion for these caregivers is paramount. Simply put, nurses must understand and respect the fundamental emotional, spiritual, and physical needs of everyone involved—the patient with dementia *and* his caregivers.

REFERENCES

Agency for Healthcare Research and Quality. (2011). *Dementia: Supporting people with dementia and their carers in health and social care.* Retrieved from https://www.ahrq.gov

American Psychiatric Association. (2013). *Diagnostic and statistical manual of mental disorders (DSM-5).* Washington, DC: American Psychiatric Association.

Bair, B., Toth, W., Johnson, M. A., Rosenberg, C., & Hurdle, J. F. (1999). Interventions for disruptive behaviors: Use and success. *Journal of Gerontological Nursing, 25*(1), 13–21.

Boyle, D. A. (2006). Delirium in older adults with cancer: Implications for practice and research. *Oncology Nursing Forum, 33*(1),61–78.

Hoe, J., Jesnick, L., Turner, R., Leavey, G., & Livingston, G. (2017). Caring for relatives with agitation at home: A qualitative study of positive coping strategies. *BJPsych Open, 3*(1), 34–40. doi: 10.1192/bjpo.bp.116.004069

Huis In Het Veld, J., Verkaik, R., van Meijel, B., Verkade, P. J., Werkman, W., Hertogh, C., & Francke, A. (2016). Self-management by family caregivers to manage changes in the behavior and mood of their relative with dementia: An online focus group study. *BMC Geriatrics, 3*(16), 95. doi: 10.1186/s12877-016-0268-4

Husebo, B. S., Achterberg, W., & Flo, E. (2016). Identifying and managing pain in people with Alzheimer's disease and other types of dementia: A systemic review. *CNS Drugs, 30*(6), 481–497. doi: 10.1007/s40263-016-0342-7

Husebo, B. S., Ballard, C., Cohen-Mansfield, J., Seifert, R., & Aarsland, D. (2014). The response of agitated behavior to pain management in persons with dementia. *American Journal of Geriatric Psychiatry, 22*(7), 708–717. doi: 10.1016/j.jagp.2012.12.006

Kales, H. C., Gitlin, L. N., Lyketsos, C. G., & Detroit Expert Panel on Assessment and Management of Neuropsychiatric Symptoms of Dementia. (2014). Management of neuropsychiatric symptoms of dementia in clinical settings: Recommendations from a multidisciplinary expert panel. *Journal of the American Geriatrics Society, 62*(4), 762–769. doi: 10.1111/jgs.12730

Keane, P. (2006). How to de-escalate potentially aggressive interactions with patients. *Synergy,* 8–10.

Kneisl, C. R., & Trigoboff, E. (2009). *Contemporary psychiatric-mental health nursing* (2nd ed.). Upper Saddle River, NJ: Prentice Hall.

Ledgerd, R., Hoe, J., Hoare, Z., Devine, M., Toot, S., Challis, D., & Orrell, M. (2016). Identifying the causes, prevention and management of crises in dementia. An online survey of stakeholders. *International Journal of Geriatric Psychiatry, 31*(6), 638–647. doi: 10.1002/gps.4371

National Institute for Health and Clinical Excellence. (2006). Dementia: Supporting people with dementia and their carers in health and social care. *NICE*. Retrieved from http://www.nice.org.uk/CG042

Power, G. A. (2010). *Dementia beyond drugs: Changing the culture of care*. Baltimore, MD: Health Professions Press.

Rueve, M. E., & Welton, R. S. (2008). Violence and mental illness. *Psychiatry, 5*(5), 34–48.

Russell-Williams, J., Jaroudi, W., Perich, T., Hoscheidt, S., El Haj, M., & Moustafa, A. A. (2018). Mindfulness and meditation: Treating cognitive impairment and reducing stress in dementia. *Reviews in the Neurosciences, 29*(7), 791–804. doi: 10.1515/revneuro-2017-0066

Savage, T., Crawford, I., & Nashed, Y. (2004). Decreasing assault occurrence on a psychogeriatric ward: An agitation management model. *Journal of Gerontological Nursing, 30*(5), 30–37.

Schuurmans, M. J., Duursma, S. A., & Shortridge-Baggett, L. M. (2001). Early recognition of delirium: Review of the literature. *Journal of Clinical Nursing, 10*(6), 721–729.

Townsend, M. C. (2015). *Psychiatric mental health nursing: Concepts of care in evidence-based practice* (8th ed.). Philadelphia, PA: F. A. Davis Company.

Varcarolis, E. M. (2011). *Manual of psychiatric nursing care planning: Assessment guides, diagnoses, psychopharmacology* (4th ed.). New York, NY: Elsevier Health Sciences.

Woods, D. L., Rapp, C. G., & Beck, C. (2004). Escalation/de-escalation patterns of behavioral symptoms of persons with dementia. *Aging & Mental Health, 8*(2), 126–132.

DE-ESCALATION OF PATIENTS WITH DELIRIUM

"Those who are free of resentful thoughts surely find peace."
–Buddha

OBJECTIVES

- Examine the origins of delirium

- Find out how to assess patients who are cognitively impaired

- Describe how to prevent escalation with the cognitively impaired

- Delineate de-escalation practices for the cognitively impaired

- Discuss how the patient's family can help

- Explore how to ensure the safety of cognitively impaired patients

Cognition is defined as the innate ability to think and reason (Townsend, 2015). Cognitive impairments result in alterations in a person's perception of reality and difficulties with communication. This can lead to situations in which de-escalation is necessary for safety.

One common type of cognitive impairment is delirium. The *DSM-5* describes *delirium* as a mental state characterized by a decreased ability to direct, focus, maintain, and shift attention (American Psychiatric Association [APA], 2013). A reduced awareness of the immediate environment, impaired memory, and difficulties with logical reasoning are other indicators of delirium. This disturbance in cognitive impairment represents a change from usual mental functions.

Delirium generally manifests as confusion, excitement, disorientation, misperceptions of reality (including illusions or visual misinterpretations, and hallucinations), or a clouding of consciousness (Twamley et al., 2002). Some patients with delirium may also experience a loss of inhibition (Oh, Fong, Hshieh, & Inouye, 2017; Stuart & Sundeen, 1991). Behaviors associated with delirium include fluctuating levels of awareness, restlessness, agitation, aggression, delusions, disorganized thought processes, and impaired judgment and decision-making.

Delirium usually develops over a short period of time, from a few hours to several days. The course of delirium is brief, from one week to one month. The severity of delirium may fluctuate throughout the day, depending on the underlying cause.

Delirium is a common psychiatric illness among medically compromised patients. Often it is a direct physiological consequence of another medical condition. It may also be a result of substance intoxication or withdrawal, of exposure to a toxin, or a combination of these factors. Delirium is usually reversible—especially with early recognition and treatment, as well as treatment of the underlying medical condition causing the delirium (APA, 2013). However, because of delirium's association with other medical illnesses, its presence can be a harbinger of significant mortality and morbidity.

> ☑ **NOTE** The prevalence of delirium is 1% to 2%. Although delirium can affect any age group, risk increases with age, rising to 14% in individuals over age 85. Delirium is most prevalent among hospitalized older adults: between 10% and 30% in emergency departments, where it often indicates an untreated medical illness (APA, 2013).

ORIGINS OF DELIRIUM

There are multiple stressors that affect brain function and may cause delirium. Some of these are hypoxias from medical conditions listed in Table 14.1.

TABLE 14.1 Medical Conditions Associated With Delirium

Anemia	Hypercarbia	Blood loss
Iron deficiencies	Folic acid deficiency	Vitamin B-12 deficiency
Dehydration	Hyperthermia	Hypothermia
Chronic obstructive pulmonary disease (COPD)	Asthma	Acute respiratory tract infection
Congestive heart failure (CHF)	Increased intercranial pressure (ICP)	Stroke
Arteriosclerosis	Hypotension	Hypertension
Subdural hematoma	Hepatic Encephalopathy	Hydrocephalus
Hypothyroidism	Hyperthyroidism	Hypoglycemia
Hypopituitarism	Adrenal disease	Malignancies

Here are other possible origins of delirium:

- Postoperative states (Townsend, 2015)

- Infectious agent such as neurosyphilis or HIV infection.

- Internal toxins from renal failure or external toxins from poisonous substances, toxic waste, or heavy metals

- Structural abnormalities such as brain tumors, brain abscess, or trauma to the brain (such as from a head injury)

- Lesions on the brain resulting in scarring (Stuart & Sundeen, 1991; Townsend, 2015)

- Nonspecific stressors such as biochemical imbalances, acetylcholine deficiencies, or use of reality-distorting drugs

ASSESSING PATIENTS WITH DELIRIUM

A comprehensive assessment of delirium involves detecting signs and symptoms of the cognitive disorder. These include the following:

- Fluctuating levels of consciousness (the main symptom of delirium)

- Disorientation

- Severe confusion (particularly at night; patient may be coherent during morning hours)

- An impaired ability to reason

- An impaired ability to engage in goal-directed behavior

- An impaired attention span

- Alternating states of hyperactivity and hypersomnolence

- Disturbance in sleep-wake cycle (e.g., daytime sleepiness, nighttime wakefulness, nighttime agitation, difficulty falling asleep, or a complete reversal of the night-day sleep-wake cycle)

- Vivid dreams and nightmares

- Intense fear or anxiety (APA, 2013; Varcarolis, 2011)

- An impairment in short-term memory

- Language disturbances (such as incoherent speech)

- Perceptual disturbances (such as hallucinations or illusions) (Marshall & Soucy, 2003)

- Aggressive or combative behavior

PREVENTING ESCALATION OF PATIENTS WITH DELIRIUM

Here are some effective practices to prevent escalation of patients with delirium:

- **Build a positive relationship.** Take time to establish a trusting relationship with patients (Boyle, 2006; Stuart & Sundeen, 1991). This can help them feel more comfortable and secure in their environment and reduce the likelihood of agitation or aggression.

- **Inform patients that their condition is short term and will improve.** This will help calm any fears patients may have about their cognitive impairment.

- **Encourage self-care and independence.** Encourage patients to do as much for themselves as they can. For example, if patients can comb their own hair, allow them to do so. Independence and self-reliance are needed life skills. They also help patients build self-esteem and self-respect.

- **Educate patients on coping skills.** These might include using verbal or written reminders to compensate for failing memory (Petersen & Negash, 2008; Tabet & Howard, 2009).

- **Identify patients' interests and skills.** Then provide adequate opportunities for patients to use them (Bartels et al., 2002).

- **Encourage patients to interact with others.** This helps restore social skills, thereby improving cognition and behavior.

- **Provide a calm environment.** A stable and quiet environment will help prevent over-excitement and agitation and help patients heal and recover.

- **Prepare patients for potentially stressful situations.** Teach patients to deal with these situations or how to avoid them in the future.

- **Provide a schedule of daily activities and procedures.** This will help the patients prepare for the day.

> **? TIP** If patients refuse to attend an activity or procedure, let a few minutes pass, and then ask them again to attend (Boyle, 2006; Stuart & Sundeen, 1991). This brief delay gives them a chance to calm down and perhaps view the proposed endeavor in a totally different light.

Restoring Optimal Memory Functioning

People suffering from delirium can benefit from interventions to improve memory functioning. This helps prevent frustration and agitated behavior. Aids to improve memory and retention include the following:

- **Place a calendar in the patient's room.** A calendar provides a concrete reminder of the current date and day of the week and keeps the patient informed of what activities may be taking place that day.

- **Place a clock in the patient's room.** Clocks are an excellent visual aid for patients, helping to remind them of the passing of time (Oh et al., 2017; Toman, 2008).

- **Hang seasonal decorations.** This will help the patient remember the time of year.

- **Display photos of loved ones in the patient's room.** This helps the patient remember who's who. (A photo album can serve the same purpose.) (Boyle, 2006; Kneisl & Trigoboff, 2009).

> ■ **Bring in items from home.** Ask a family member to bring items from home for placement in the patient's room. This will make the patient's surroundings feel more familiar.
>
> ■ **Display items related to the patient's hobbies or interests.** These can serve as cues to jog the patient's memory.
>
> These objects can help calm and comfort the patient until the delirium lifts.

DE-ESCALATION TECHNIQUES FOR PATIENTS WITH DELIRIUM

If patients with delirium becomes aggressive, try these de-escalation techniques:

■ **Validate patients' feelings.** For example, say, "I know you are upset because your brother has not arrived yet to visit." This conveys that you understand the situation and that you care.

■ **Divert patients.** If the patient's brother is late, try saying, "Tell me about your brother." This has the added benefit of providing the patient with an opportunity to reminisce about the family member (in other words, to engage in reminiscence therapy—see the next bullet).

■ **Engage patients in reminiscence therapy.** This can help patients to cope with their cognitive deficits and restore calm behavior.

■ **Reorient patients.** Make patients aware of the date and time and their location.

■ **Reassure patients that they are safe.** Tell patients where they are and that they are safe. This reassurance can comfort and calm delirious patients with fluctuating awareness.

■ **Discourage delusional thinking.** Don't feed into patients' hallucinations or delusions by appearing to validate made-up stories or suggesting that you see something that is not there. Instead, gently correct patients and redirect them to real events and real people. For example, say, "I know you say a person is standing in the doorway, but I do not see anyone there," and direct them back to what is present and real.

■ **Play music.** Music can have an especially calming effect on agitated individuals who are cognitively impaired. Music reduces muscle tension and anxiety and stimulates memory (Cheong, 2004; Cohen-Mansfield, 2004). For patients suffering from delirium, music can also improve mood and behavior. Music with no words and a slow tempo is best.

> **? TIP** Some patients suffering from delirium tend to wander. For these patients, it's best to walk with them for a while before gently redirecting them back to their room.

Guidelines for Communicating With Patients Experiencing Delirium

■ **Approach the patient from the front.** Approaching from behind could startle the patient, causing agitation or aggression. Also, speak to the patient face to face.

■ **Keep things short and simple.** Be clear and direct (Chertkow et al., 2008; Marshall & Soucy, 2003). This makes it more likely you'll receive an appropriate response and helps the patient maintain self-control.

■ **Keep choices to a minimum.** Although it's good to give patients choices, too many choices can overwhelm patients who are cognitively impaired.

■ **Use alternative modes of communication.** For example, use text, pictures, hand gestures, pantomime, or role play to get your message across (Boyle, 2006; Varcarolis, 2011).

■ **Give praise.** Recognize patients when they exercise their better-preserved abilities or hit important milestones. This helps raise the patient's self-respect and self-esteem.

■ **Ask open-ended questions.** This encourages the patient to communicate thoughts and feelings.

■ **Explain procedures.** Patients with cognitive impairment such as delirium may become agitated when they are made to do something new or unfamiliar. To prevent this, step them through any activities or procedures you want them to complete, and explain your expectations.

■ **Don't over-promise.** If you can't deliver on a promise to a patient with delirium, don't make it.

■ **Speak to the patient on an adult level.** Don't talk down to the patient.

TEST YOURSELF

DELIRIUM Mrs. Alexander is a 74-year-old retired librarian whose daughter, Ellen, has brought her to the emergency department (ED). Mrs. Alexander is incoherent and confused upon arrival.

Ellen provides her mother's medical history. Ellen says that Mrs. Alexander had no prior illness or prescription medications ordered. She explains that her mother lives alone and has always been alert and oriented to reality. Ellen says that recently she has noticed a change in her mother's normal habits. She says that her mother had begun having problems sleeping and has started taking an over-the-counter sleep aid purchased at the corner pharmacy without consulting her physician.

Ellen says she received a call this morning from Mrs. Alexander's neighbor. The neighbor told Ellen that Mrs. Alexander was walking semi-clothed and barefoot in her front yard in freezing temperatures. Ellen hurried to her mother's home. When she arrived, she found Mrs. Alexander indoors. "Who are you?" Mrs. Alexander screamed at Ellen, shaking her fists at her daughter. "Why are you in my house?" Mrs. Alexander then pointed at a medication bottle on the table and began repeating over and over, "This new medicine is making me sick!" Ellen checked the medicine bottle. It was her mother's sleeping medication. Ellen discovered the bottle was empty despite Mrs. Alexander having purchased it just three days prior.

At the ED, Mrs. Alexander is assessed and transferred to an inpatient medical unit. All medications are placed on hold and intravenous hydration is started. Mrs. Alexander remains confused and disoriented to person, place, time, and situation, however. She is agitated. "I see fish flying around!" she shouts.

How would you handle this situation?

WORKING WITH FAMILY MEMBERS

Involving the patient's family members, such as a significant other, in the patient's care can help the patient cope with the stresses associated with the condition (Marshall & Soucy, 2003; Tabet & Howard, 2009). Family members can also help facilitate communication and share the patient's habits and preferences.

As a first step, educate the patient and family members about the nature of the problem and the recommended healthcare plan. As care proceeds, meet regularly with family members to update them and provide them with an opportunity to talk. Finally, involve the patient and family in discharge planning. Maintaining these caring relationships with others promotes a positive self-concept and motivates the patient to reorient to reality and demonstrate appropriate behavior.

ENSURING THE SAFETY OF PATIENTS WITH DELIRIUM

Delirium usually involves an impairment of the senses and of perception that can endanger patients' safety. When caring for patients with delirium, you'll need to take special steps to ensure they stay safe. These include the following:

- **Ensure the patients have access to needed sensory aids such as eyeglasses and hearing aids.** These sensory aids improve patient safety by preventing falls (Boyle, 2006). They also allow for improved perception of sight and sound, which help reorient the patients to reality.

- **Ensure the patients have access to ambulatory aids.** If the patients have an unsteady gait, make sure they have access to a cane or walker.

- **Stay alert.** With some delirious patients, one-to-one observation may be necessary for safety.

- **Place the patients in a room near the nurse's station.** This allows for closer and more frequent observation.

- **Remove safety hazards.** These could include pathway obstacles, spills on the floor, open flames (such as with matches or other fire-ignition devices), or inadequate lighting (Stuart & Sundeen, 1991).

- **Protect them from injury.** During periods of confusion, protect the patients from injury by assisting with ambulation to prevent falls, providing a well-lighted room, and providing assistance with any activities of daily living.

REFERENCES

American Psychiatric Association. (2013). *Diagnostic and statistical manual of mental disorders (DSM-5)*. Washington, DC: American Psychiatric Association.

Bartels, S. J., Dums, A. R., Oxman, T. E., Schneider, L. S., Aréan, P. A., Alexopoulos, G. S., & Jeste, D. V. (2002). Evidence-based practices in geriatric mental health care. *Psychiatric Services, 53*(11), 1,419–1,431.

Boyle, D. A. (2006). Delirium in older adults with cancer: Implications for practice and research. *Oncology Nursing Forum, 33*(1), 61–78.

Cheong, J. A. (2004). An evidence-based approach to the management of agitation in the geriatric patient. *Focus, 2*(2), 197–205.

Chertkow, H., Massoud, F., Nasreddine, Z., Belleville, S., Joanette, Y., Bocti, C., … Bergman, H. (2008). Diagnosis and treatment of dementia: 3. Mild cognitive impairment and cognitive impairment without dementia. *Canadian Medical Association Journal, 178*(10), 1,273–1,285. doi: 10.1503/cmaj.070797

Cohen-Mansfield, J. (2004). Nonpharmacologic interventions for inappropriate behaviors in dementia: A review, summary, and critique. *The American Journal of Geriatric Psychiatry, 9*(4), 361–381.

Kneisl, C. R., & Trigoboff, E. (2009). *Contemporary psychiatric-mental health nursing* (2nd ed.). Upper Saddle River, NJ: Prentice Hall.

Marshall, M. C., & Soucy, M. D. (2003). Delirium in the intensive care unit. *Critical Care Nursing Quarterly, 26*(3), 172–178.

Oh, E. S., Fong, T. G., Hshieh, T. T., Inouye, S. K. (2017). Delirium in older persons: Advances in diagnosis and treatment, *JAMA, 318*(12), 1,161–1,174. doi: 10.1001/jama.2017.12067

Petersen, R. C., & Negash, S. (2008). Mild cognitive impairment: An overview. *CNS Spectrums, 13*(1), 45–53.

Stuart, G. W., & Sundeen, S. J. (1991). *Principles and practice of psychiatric nursing* (4th ed.). St. Louis, MO: Mosby.

Tabet, N., & Howard, R. (2009). Non-pharmacological interventions in the prevention of delirium. *Age and Ageing, 38*(4), 374–379. doi: 10.1093/ageing/afp039

Toman, B. (2008). The science of healthy aging. *Mayo Clinic,* 1–3.

Townsend, M. C. (2015). *Psychiatric mental health nursing: Concepts of care in evidence-based practice* (8th ed.). Philadelphia, PA: F. A. Davis Company.

Twamley, E. W., Doshi, R. R., Nayak, G. V., Palmer, B. W., Golshan, S., Heaton, R. K., … Jeste, D. V. (2002). Generalized cognitive impairments, ability to perform everyday tasks, and level of independence in community living situations of older patients with psychosis. *The American Journal of Psychiatry, 159*(12), 2,013–2,020.

Varcarolis, E. M. (2011). *Manual of psychiatric nursing care planning: Assessment guides, diagnoses, psychopharmacology* (4th ed.). New York, NY: Elsevier Health Sciences.

15

DE-ESCALATION OF "DIFFICULT" PATIENTS

"Peace in ourselves, peace in the world."
–Thích Nhất Hạnh

OBJECTIVES

- Examine the origins of difficult behavior
- Find out how to assess difficult patients
- Describe de-escalation practices for difficult patients
- Find out how to help difficult patients who are elderly

Every nurse or healthcare provider has at one time or another encountered a "difficult" patient. There is no single definition of what constitutes difficult behavior, however. Indeed, the term *difficult* is used to describe a range of patients. These include the following:

- **Indecisive patients.** These patients take hours to make a decision and keep changing their mind.

- **Complainers.** These patients complain about everything at every opportunity, from the food, to the TV channel, to every aspect of their immediate care.

- **Silent patients.** These patients refuse to verbalize any of their problems, issues, or needs—bottling up their emotions until they finally explode in a torrent of rage.

- **Aggressive patients.** These patients are generally disagreeable or argumentative.

- **Negativists.** These patients do the opposite of any instructions received and refuse every care request, complicating their own care.

Regardless of whether a patient is indecisive, complaining, or some other form of difficult, all difficult patients have certain behaviors in common. For example, difficult patients often (Juliana et al., 1997):

- Demand special privileges that others do not receive

- Frequently make insulting remarks toward others

- Violate facility rules

- Act helpless

- Fail to cooperate with requests

- Play staff members against each other to cause tension among the team (known as *staff-splitting*)

- Fail to comply with treatment regimens

- Use threats rather than requests to get their needs met

- Hold up the flow of work by making unnecessary demands, complaining, or refusing to cooperate

> ☑ **NOTE** Basically, the "difficult" label is applied to patients who consume more time than is normally necessary for their care or engage in some level of refusal or nonadherence to care instructions.

Difficult patients often share certain characteristics, too—although with varying levels of intensity (Juliana et al., 1997; Wolf & Robinson-Smith, 2007). (See Table 15.1.)

TABLE 15.1 Characteristics of the Difficult Patient

Demanding	Deceptive	Aggressive	Angry
Violent	Frightened	Recalcitrant	Staff-splitting
Dependent	Threatening	Disinhibited	Insulting
Confused	Sexually inappropriate	Moody	Bullying
Irrational	Attention seeking	Self-harming	Easily agitated
Poor hygiene	Poor care adherence	Manipulative	Rude

De-escalating difficult patients can be a challenge—but it's one that all nurses and other caregivers must meet. All human beings are worthy of respect, care, and compassion—even difficult patients. Besides, with patience and understanding, you might just convert that difficult patient into a dream charge.

ORIGINS OF DIFFICULT BEHAVIORS

Ultimately, patients exhibit difficult behavior for various reasons. Here are just a few possibilities:

- Pain or discomfort
- Stress or grief due to the loss of a loved one
- Fear
- Feelings of hopelessness or worthlessness
- Poor coping skills
- A tendency to bottle up emotion until the patient explodes
- Reaction to medication

Research indicates that patient care groups most closely associated with difficult behavior are those with chronic pain, complex care issues, substance abuse, chronic fatigue syndrome, obsessive compulsive disorder, or addictive disorders (Brunero, Fairbrother, Lee, & Davis, 2007; Macdonald, 2003).

Mental illness is another contributor. Prevalence studies have found patients who are identified as difficult are twice as likely to suffer from mental illness. For example, major psychiatric illnesses such as schizophrenia and bipolar disorder are significant causes of difficult behavior. The following psychiatric diagnoses may also be linked to difficult behavior (Koekkoek, van Meijel, & Hutschemaekers, 2006):

- **Psychotic disorders.** These types of disorders distort thought processes, which can trigger difficult behavior.

- **Personality disorders.** These include borderline personality disorder, narcissistic personality disorder, and antisocial personality disorder. Patients with these disorders lack emotional control, have an inflated sense of self-esteem, and exhibit aberrant social behaviors, respectively—all drivers of difficult behavior.

- **Chronic depression.** Manifestations of chronic depression such as irritability, low frustration tolerance, and decreased energy can lead to difficult behavior.

- **Schizoid and schizotypal conditions.** Because these conditions involve a distorted perception of reality, they commonly cause difficult behavior.

> ☑ **NOTE** Understanding why some patients are difficult, and using therapeutic communication techniques to defuse difficult behavior, can help nurses develop a therapeutic working relationship with the patient (Nettina, 2010).

ASSESSING A DIFFICULT PATIENT

When assessing a difficult patient, be alert for behavioral signs or body language that may indicate escalation. These might include the following:

- Agitated motion

- Loud or profane speech

- A clenched jaw or fist

- A flushed face

- Enlarged eyes

- Flared nostrils

- Rapid breathing

A thorough assessment also involves observing for signs of imminent violent behavior such as the following:

- Verbal threats

- Demands for immediate attention

- Encroaching on another's personal space

> **⚠ CAUTION** As always, early assessment and intervention is critical.

PREVENTING ESCALATION WITH DIFFICULT PATIENTS

With difficult patients, communicating is key to preventing escalation. Here are a few specific therapeutic communication techniques you can try. (For more on these techniques, refer to Chapter 5, "Therapeutic Communication for De-Escalation.")

- **Greet patients with their full name or use an honorific.** This conveys your respect.

- **Introduce yourself.** Use your first name, last name, and title so the patients know who you are and what your role is in their care.

- **Offer availability.** Let the patients know you are there to help.

- **Encourage patients to verbalize.** Start the conversation with an observation like, "You seem worried about something." Then ask open-ended questions such as, "What is upsetting you?" (Hosley & Molle-Matthews, 2006)

- **Don't rush patients.** Give them plenty of time to express their feelings and to answer questions (Hosley & Molle-Matthews, 2006).

- **Acknowledge that you are listening.** For example, nod your head as patients speak.

- **Make sure you understand what patients are saying.** Use therapeutic communication techniques like restating, reflecting, focusing, and questioning to ensure you're clear on the patients' message.

> ☑ **NOTE** Communicating with difficult patients can be a challenge. Still, nurses must make every effort to do so in a therapeutic manner. This requires critical thinking, patience, and diplomacy. The therapeutic healthcare professional must maintain self-control, always role modeling calm and appropriate behavior for the patient.

In addition to practicing therapeutic communication, ensuring continuity of caregivers can help prevent difficult patients from escalating. Consistently interacting with the same caregivers enables the difficult patient to build trusting relationships with healthcare staff. On a related note, you should also ensure consistency in interventions and actions among the staff (Butler, 1986; Juliana et al., 1997).

EFFECTIVE DE-ESCALATION PRACTICES FOR DIFFICULT PATIENTS

As is often the case, the most effective de-escalation technique for difficult patients is encouraging patients to talk about their issues—in other words, verbal de-escalation. Allowing patients to verbalize pent-up emotions acts as a catharsis, helps to defuse their anger or aggression, and helps them regain self-control. As difficult patients speak, listen closely to what they say to ensure that they feel heard.

As you converse with difficult patients, reflect empathy. Make them aware that you understand their situation and their feelings. Showing empathy is a primary intervention to establish therapeutic rapport with difficult patients. So too is showing caring and concern.

Offer to help the patients (Caroll, 2004). Make them clearly aware of your intention to help find a solution that is beneficial to all involved. Ask the patients what they think could be done to improve the situation. Attempt to identify their goals and what is keeping them from those goals (Butler, 1986; Juliana et al., 1997). Make the patients aware that you are doing everything in your power to help them.

Avoid arguing with the patients or engaging in a power struggle. This will only compound the issue and cause the conflict to escalate. If necessary, set limits. Calmly but firmly indicate your expectations regarding their behavior, and make them aware of your boundaries (Fishkind, 2002). This should be a nonconfrontational and respectful discussion. Remember: Only set limits that you can and will enforce.

Here are more ways to de-escalate difficult patients:

- **Encourage patients to perform relaxation exercises.** An example might be progressive muscular relaxation. This can help relieve the stress that is causing the difficult behavior (Seaward, 2006).

- **Redirect difficult patients.** Difficult patients often need more instruction than "regular" ones. Often they require a special type of redirection that involves telling them not only what they are doing wrong but how to do that thing right. For example, suppose difficult patients constantly and loudly complain that their dinner tray never has food they like. An appropriate redirection technique might be to remind them that a menu is placed in their room every day, and that if they take the time to complete it, then they will receive foods they prefer. Then say, "I will be happy to help you fill out the menu. We are here to help you." Redirecting in a respectful and courteous way will help defuse the anger often present in difficult patients.

- **Give patients choices.** This will give patients a sense of empowerment over their situation.

- **Educate patients.** Sometimes nurses are so focused on telling patients to stop an *incorrect* behavior, they forget the patients might not know the *correct* behavior. Educate patients on what behaviors they should exhibit, such as courtesy and respect for others. While you're at it, educate patients about safety, and remind them that they must act as a partner to help keep the environment safe for everyone.

Throughout the interaction, project calmness, be assertive, and be confident. This is critical when dealing with difficult patients. Patience is also key. Finally, speak slowly, and avoid abrupt movements.

Guidelines for Communicating With Difficult Patients

- *Never talk about patients like they are not present.* Always assume patients can hear and understand everything you say in front of them.

- **Speak in a normal tone.** Don't shout or raise your voice. Speaking louder does not increase comprehension.

- **Speak on an adult level.** Often, difficult patients have problems communicating. This doesn't mean they have impaired intelligence, however. It may just mean they have difficulty getting their point across. Speak to these patients as adults to avoid upsetting them further.

- **Avoid carrying on more than one conversation at a time.** Give patients your undivided attention—and make sure they give you their undivided attention, too.

- **Ask simple questions that require only short answers.** This will prevent you from overwhelming the patients.

- **Ensure the environment is quiet and relaxed.** Reduce noxious noises that might disturb or distract the patients to facilitate open communication.

- **Speak to the patients at eye level.** If patients are in wheelchairs or in their beds, sit down to talk with them. Also, maintain eye contact with the patients during the conversation.

- **Don't rush the patients.** Give them adequate time to formulate a reply, and don't interrupt the patients when they speak (Nettina, 2010).

- **Ask for clarification.** If you don't understand something the patients say, ask them to clarify it.

- **Summarize the communication.** When you're finished speaking with patients, summarize what was said to make sure you understood everything correctly.

TEST YOURSELF

THE DIFFICULT PATIENT Mr. Mitchell is a 56-year-old man who is a newly admitted inpatient at a healthcare facility. He is diabetic and suffers from bipolar disorder. Mr. Mitchell had a stroke two years ago and is unable to clearly voice his needs and feelings. Mr. Mitchell is often angry and frustrated by his inability to be clearly understood. At times, Mr. Mitchell gets angry and becomes physically aggressive with staff, often without warning.

Today Mr. Mitchell's physician has informed him that his request to be discharged has been denied. Mr. Mitchell shakes his fists and begins shouting obscenities at the physician.

How would you handle this situation?

AIDING DIFFICULT PATIENTS WHO ARE ELDERLY

When difficult patients are also elderly, you must take special care during your interactions with them and work even harder to prevent escalation.

> ✅ **NOTE** Effectively managing the behavior of difficult elderly patients requires a team approach that involves multidisciplinary domains partnering with patients, their families, and their caregivers (Paterson, Leadbetter, & McComish, 1997).

One way to prevent escalation is to avoid overwhelming elderly patients with information. Being overwhelmed causes many elderly patients to become agitated. When educating or sharing information with elderly patients, keep these points in mind:

- **Slow down your speech.** Use a steady, calm, and pleasant voice.

- **Use visual aids.** Draw pictures or diagrams or use photos to reinforce your verbal communication.

- **Provide a written copy.** When giving instructions, give patients a written copy of them to review later. This will help patients remember what you've told them.

- **Present information one item at a time.** Don't bombard patients with everything at once.

- **Repeat the information several times.** When discussing procedures, treatments, and patient interventions, repeat the relevant information several times to ensure it sinks in (Haas, Leiser, Magill, & Sanyer, 2005).

- **Role play.** This may help the information "stick." Role play can also help prepare elderly patients to handle stressful situations in the future— another way to prevent escalation.

- **Ask for feedback.** When you finish discussing one topic, ask patients for feedback to ensure they have understood before progressing to the next topic.

If your goal is to encourage elderly, difficult patients to change their behavior, be specific in the change you want to see made, and make sure the patients clearly understand what you're after. Change may occur more slowly with the elderly, but with education and motivation, it is possible.

REFERENCES

Brunero, S., Fairbrother, G., Lee, S., & Davis, M. (2007). Clinical characteristics of people with mental health problems who frequently attend an Australian emergency department. *Australian Health Review, 31*(3), 462–470.

Butler, B. M. (1986). When a nurse and patient battle for control. *RN, 49*(9), 67–68.

Caroll, V. (2004). Preventing violence in the healthcare workplace. *The Alabama Nurse, 31*(1), 23.

Fishkind, A. (2002). Calming agitation with words, not drugs: 10 commandments for safety. *Current Psychiatry, 1*(4), 32–39.

Haas, L. J., Leiser, J. P., Magill, M. K., & Sanyer, O. N. (2005). Management of the difficult patient. *American Family Physician, 72*(10), 2,063–2,068.

Hosley, J., & Molle-Matthews, E. (2006). *A practical guide to therapeutic communication for healthcare professionals.* St. Louis, MO: Saunders.

Juliana, C. A, Orehowsky, S., Smith-Regojo, P., Sikora, S. M., Smith, P. A., Stein, D. K., … Wolf, Z. R. (1997). Interventions used by staff to manage "difficult" patients. *Holistic Nursing Practice, 11*(4), 1–26.

Koekkoek, B., van Meijel, B., & Hutschemaekers, G. (2006). "Difficult patients" in mental health care: A review. *Psychiatric Services, 57*(6), 795–802.

Macdonald, M. (2003). Seeing the cage: Stigma and its potential to inform the concept of the difficult patient. *Clinical Nurse Specialist, 17*(6), 305–310.

Nettina, S. M. (2010). *Lippincott manual of nursing practice* (9th ed.). Philadelphia, PA: Lippincott Williams & Wilkins.

Paterson, B., Leadbetter, D., & McComish, A. (1997). De-escalation in the management of aggression and violence. *Nursing Times, 93*(36), 58–61.

Seaward, B. L. (2012). *Managing stress: Principles and strategies for health and well-being* (7th ed.). Burlington, VT: Jones & Bartlett Learning.

Wolf, Z. R., & Robinson-Smith, G. (2007). Strategies used by clinical nurse specialists in "difficult" clinician-patient situations. *Clinical Nurse Specialist, 21*(2), 74–84.

DE-ESCALATION OF ANGRY PATIENTS

"For every minute you remain angry,
you give up 60 seconds of peace of mind."
–Ralph Waldo Emerson

OBJECTIVES

- Identify types of expressions of anger

- Examine the origins of anger and common anger triggers

- Find out how to prevent patients from expressing anger inappropriately

- Explore de-escalation techniques for angry patients

Anger is defined as a strong, unpleasant, and uncomfortable emotional response to an unwanted provocation resulting from injury, mistreatment, or opposition (Schiraldi & Kerr, 2002). In our stress-filled culture, anger is everywhere. Television shows, movies, and music are packed with expressions of anger. Indeed, there is so much anger in our world today, future historians may well refer to this era as the "age of anger."

Anger is a normal human emotion. In fact, it is a self-protective survival instinct. Only when anger goes out of bounds does it become dysfunctional—sometimes destroying families, careers, and communities. Although anger cannot be eliminated from the human experience, it *can* be managed and controlled (Edwards & Loprinzi, 2018; Maiuro, 1987). Part of anger management is de-escalating anger—in ourselves and in others. That's the focus of this chapter.

TYPES OF EXPRESSIONS OF ANGER

There are two types of expressions of anger: negative and positive. Negative expressions of anger come in various forms. One form is self-destructive anger. Examples of negative self-destructive angry behaviors include (Kassinove & Tafrate, 2002):

- Negative self-talk—for example, "You are so stupid. No one will ever love you!"

- Taking everything personally

- Assuming others are upset with them instead of listening to prevent misunderstandings

- Excessive alcohol use

- Taking drugs

- Reckless driving

- Looking for fights

- Feeling outraged for even the most minor slight.

> ☑ **NOTE** Negative self-talk also includes self-talk meant to escalate your anger, such as, "He hurt me on purpose!" or, "I'll get her back!" These negative expressions of anger can cause an escalation in aggression or even violence.

Another form of negative anger is uncontrolled rage—the kind that often explodes into violence. This type of out-of-control anger can result in very negative consequences, such as the following:

- Physical harm to yourself, a loved one, or others

- Diminished physical or mental health (Nolan et al., 2003)

- The destruction of property (which may bring with it significant legal and financial repercussions)

- The loss of relationships with family members or friends

- A poor reputation

- The loss of a career

- The loss of social privileges

- Jail time (Kassinove & Tafrate, 2002; Morland et al., 2010)

In contrast, positive expressions of anger are constructive. Examples of positive expressions of anger include airing grievances so they can be addressed immediately and problem-solving to address the issue that is causing the anger. Positive expressions of anger can also drive change meant to prevent people from feeling angry in the future. For example, addicts could become so angry about their addiction, they could decide to become clean and sober (Shorey, McNulty, Moore, & Stuart, 2017).

> ✅ **NOTE** Sobriety is a beneficial outcome of positive expressions of anger. It can change lives for the better.

Just as there's such a thing as negative self-talk, there's positive self-talk. This can empower the individual to make a change for a better life. The most-high impact instances of self-talk use "I" statements to describe feelings, define desired changes in behavior, or demonstrate self-love or caring (Boyd, 2008). For example (Kassinove & Tafrate, 2002):

- "I am in control of my emotions."

- "I accept and acknowledge my emotions."

- "I can learn to express my anger in beneficial ways."

- "I express angry emotions in ways that are caring toward myself and others."

- "I can change for the better."

ORIGINS OF ANGER AND COMMON ANGER TRIGGERS

Scientists have developed four main theories for the origins of anger in humans:

- **Psychoanalytic theory.** This is the theory that emotions such as anger are psychological and instinctual and that suppressing these emotions is unhealthy to one's mental health.

- **Biologic theory.** This theory proposes that major causes of anger are biological. For example, biological factors such as neurochemical triggers, developmental deficits, anoxia, malnutrition, toxins, tumors, and neurodegenerative diseases cause or contribute to anger (Edwards & Loprinzi, 2018).

- **Behavioral theory.** According to this theory, anger is a learned response to a specific stimulus.

- **Sociocultural theory.** This theory suggests that anger originates from cultural influences of high-pressure, high-stress, competitive, and success-oriented environments (Boyd, 2008).

Regardless of its origins in the human species, anger begins when an individual becomes overloaded with stress. Stressors that commonly spark anger include:

- Emotional stress, such as from a breakup with a spouse or significant other

- Financial problems (especially stressful following the recent economic downturn in which many people lost their livelihoods and families lost their homes)

- Personal conflicts

- Unpleasant events or reminders, such as the anniversary of the death of a loved one

- Unpleasant memories—for example, of physical or emotional harm

- Excessive use of alcohol or substance abuse (Edwards & Loprinzi, 2018)

- Medical health issues that cause pain or emotional turmoil

- Work-related stress

- Perceived threats to one's way of life or livelihood

> ☑ **NOTE** If you encounter angry patients while working in a healthcare facility, be aware that the facility and its staff are likely *not* the source of that anger. Although the patients' anger might be directed at the healthcare staff, it is most likely caused by the situation in which the individuals find themselves or the emotional stress they are experiencing as a result of that situation.

The Pattern of Anger

Anger often follows a fairly predictable pattern:

1. It begins with a stressor—either internal or external.

2. After the stressor is felt, anxiety and tension build.

3. With no outlet available, the person starts to become angry.

4. As anger builds, physiologic changes occur. The heart races, the blood pressure rises, and the stomach becomes tight or upset. The person may also clench fists and jaw, become flushed, feel pressure on the temples, have sweaty palms, or feel hot or breathless, especially as respirations increase (Maier, Stava, Morrow, van Rybroek, & Bauman, 1987).

5. As the intensity of the anger grows, the person may experience the fight-or-flight instinct. (This was discussed in more detail in Chapter 6, "Stress-Management Techniques.")

How the person responds in this situation determines whether the anger is normal or dysfunctional. This is the vicious cycle of anger.

ASSESSING THE ANGRY PATIENT

The expression of anger both inwardly and outwardly toward others has many origins. A nurse's primary goal when assessing an angry patient is to identify any function or secondary gain that anger, frustration, or rage may provide for the individual, as well as other causes.

Anger can be a learned behavior—one that begins in childhood when a parent says "no," and the child throws a tantrum and then gets his or her way. Nurses should assess whether the patient is receiving some type of external reward for angry behavior. Patients can also learn dysfunctional anger from negative role models in childhood. Finally, anger can arise from biological causes such as hormonal dysfunction or from interactions with the environment such as from crowding.

In addition to assessing whether the patient is expressing anger, the nurse should determine whether the patient has difficulty regulating or controlling anger when it arises.

PREVENTING PATIENTS FROM EXPRESSING ANGER INAPPROPRIATELY

Nurses can help patients develop healthy strategies to express their anger in more positive ways. This is called anger management. Anger management involves using learned skills to respond appropriately to anger through self–de-escalation (Aboulafia-Brakha & Ptak, 2016).

With anger management, an individual who struggles to control anger is taught how to recognize triggers for anger, identify common symptoms of anger, consider potential consequences of anger, and respond in a normal manner by using de-escalation techniques to break the anger cycle (Aboulafia-Brakha & Ptak, 2016). Internal cues of feelings of anger are explored, as are coping mechanisms to deal with angry feelings without a loss of self-control.

To start, explain to the patient the holistic benefits of expressing anger appropriately and nonviolently (Goldstein et al, 2018; Walitzer, Deffenbacher, & Shyhalla, 2015). Also convey your belief that the patient is capable of controlling the behavior. With that out of the way, you can assist the patient to develop appropriate ways to express anger—for example, calmly stating the problem that is upsetting rather than acting out in anger.

> **? TIP** Help the patient identify "anger role models"—that is, people who express anger appropriately. Even better, be that role model yourself.

Another technique is to encourage the patient to use cognitive restructuring to alter any irrational thoughts that might be fueling anger as well as any maladaptive behaviors that might prevent problem-solving, such as accusing, attacking, or catastrophizing. (*Catastrophizing* is blowing everything out of proportion by thinking that only the worst will happen without considering the more likely possibility of positive outcomes.) Sometimes it is a person's negative *perception* of a situation that triggers the anger response; cognitive restructuring involves learning to consider the situation in a new, healthier, and more positive way. For example, suppose a person (let's call him Bob) begins to feel judged by another person (let's call him Theo) with whom he is conversing. Instead of becoming angry, Bob could choose to look at the situation in a different light (Schiraldi & Kerr, 2002). Bob could say to himself, "Maybe Theo is in a bad mood because of his own personal problems," or "Maybe he just had an argument with his wife and he is upset with her, not me." Simply put, cognitive restructuring allows for a more rational perspective on the situation and identifies possible wrong assumptions, which prevents feelings of anger from presenting themselves.

Finally, teach the patient to use calming measures such as mental imagery, meditation, deep breathing, physical exercise, or progressive muscular relaxation (PMR) to relieve anger, anxiety, and tension (Boyd, 2008; Edwards & Loprinzi, 2018; Maiuro, 1987; Petruzzello, Landers, Hatfield, Kubitz, & Salazar, 1991; Seaward, 2012; Tang, Hölzel, & Posner, 2015). For more on these techniques, refer to Chapter 6. Or, have the patient employ a time-out strategy—counting to ten before reacting.

> **? TIP**   Praise patients when they express anger in an appropriate way to provide positive reinforcement.

Lewin's Change Model

Lewin's (1951) change model can be applied to anger management and serve as a beneficial model of behavioral change. The stages of this model are as follows:

1. **Preparing to change.** In this stage, the person conducts a self-assessment. This often brings a new awareness of experiences involving anger and of anger's impact on the self and others. It also conveys an increasing motivation to change how the person expresses anger. The individual develops a strong therapeutic alliance during this phase.

2. **Changing.** In this phase, the person learns to avoid anger triggers or to react to them differently—for example, walking away from an argument rather than exploding in anger. This phase also involves building life skills that relate to self-control and problem-solving to avoid the escalation of anger. Examples of these life skills might include relaxation exercises (such as deep breathing) or cognitive restructuring. Finally, this phase involves forgiveness—of others and of the self. Forgiveness means

continues

releasing past hurts and resentments to bring peace in the future. Holding grudges only feeds aberrant anger; when we forgive, we can let that anger go. The final test of this phase is exposure to an anger catalyst to verify the person's ability to maintain self-control.

3. **Maintaining change.** In this stage, the change has occurred. The person can now maintain self-control in the face of anger. So, preventing a re-occurrence of the old, out-of-control behaviors is the primary concern here (Kassinove & Tafrate, 2002). The person maintains the change by practicing the change until it comes naturally.

DE-ESCALATION TECHNIQUES FOR ANGRY PATIENTS

When facing an angry person, there are several interventional techniques you can use to de-escalate the situation. As always, it's critical to intervene as early as possible, and if the person directs anger toward himself or others, you must take steps to ensure the safety of all involved to prevent physical harm (Boyd, 2008; Petruzzello et al., 1991).

Encouraging the person to verbalize—for example, by asking open-ended questions—is key. (Refer to Chapter 5, "Therapeutic Communication for De-Escalation," for information on how best to achieve this.) This can help you establish trust and rapport with the patient. Take a calm, caring, and reassuring approach, and remain aware of yourself, your appearance, and your demeanor.

If the person is angry with someone else (rather than because of a negative situation), recommend approaching that person directly to discuss the issue. Try to help both parties see the situation in a more positive manner, identify ways to defuse the anger, and reach agreement. (For more information on helping parties resolve conflict, refer to Chapter 7, "Conflict Resolution.") If the individual who provoked the person's anger is not available, suggest the person discuss the anger with a trusted friend or family member. This can help to defuse the angry feelings (Boyd, 2008; Shorey, Seavey, Quinn, & Cornelius, 2014).

For more suggested interventions, see Table 16.1.

TABLE 16.1 Anger Management and De-Escalation Interventions

Reduce stressors	Exercise daily	Eat well-balanced meals	Meditate
Sleep well	Verbalize issues	Listen to music	Find self-awareness
Recognize anger triggers	Journal/write	Walk/jog	Enjoy quiet time
Take a time out (count to ten before reacting)	Engage in positive self-talk	Seek entertainment	Think before acting
Laugh	Forgive	Use progressive muscular relaxation	Do yoga

CASE STUDY

ANGER MANAGEMENT

Gary is a 23-year-old male inpatient in a medical facility for cancer treatment. Gary is pacing back and forth in his room, pounding his fist into his palm in an angry rage. This is unusual, as earlier, Gary was in a good mood and was very cooperative. The nurse approaches Gary to try to de-escalate the situation.

Nurse: Gary, you seem angry. What has happened to make you so upset?

Gary: Yesterday, the oncologist said I would be discharged tomorrow, but today I was told that discharge won't be until Thursday.

Nurse: I know sometimes patients get upset when their discharge is cancelled. Is that how you feel?

Gary: Yes! The oncologist should not have promised me a discharge if there was uncertainty. I feel cheated!

Nurse: It sounds like this experience is making you feel disappointed.

Gary: I feel very disappointed. I promised to attend a birthday party tomorrow night, and now I can't go. Everyone is trying to control me. I have no say-so in my life anymore. When I am treated this way, I start to get angry, and it gets worse and worse until I break something!

Nurse: Gary, your doctor will be coming by to see you tomorrow at 7 a.m., right after your scheduled blood test. Would you like for me to be here with you then?

Gary: That would be great! I get all tongue-tied when I am upset. I can't talk right sometimes.

Nurse: I can't make any promises as to what you'll be told, but I will be here when you speak with the doctor. In the meantime, would you like to learn some deep-breathing exercises to help you relax until the doctor gets here?

Gary: Yes! Thanks. I would really like that. It's great to know you are here to help me!

REFERENCES

Aboulafia-Brakha, T., & Ptak, R. (2016). Effects of group psychotherapy on anger management following acquired brain injury. *Brain Injury, 30*(9), 1,121–1,130. doi: 10.1080/02699052.2016.1174784

Boyd, M. A. (2008). *Psychiatric nursing: Contemporary practice* (4th ed.). Philadelphia, PA: Lippincott, Williams & Wilkins.

Edwards, M. K., & Loprinzi, P. D. (2018). Experimental effects of brief, single bouts of walking and meditation on mood profile in young adults. *Health Promotion Perspectives, 8*(3), 171–178. doi: 10.15171/hpp.2018.23

Goldstein, N. E. S., Giallella, C. L., Haney-Caron, E., Peterson, L., Serico, J., Kemp, K., ... Lochman, J. (2018). Juvenile Justice Anger Management (JJAM) Treatment for girls: Results of a randomized controlled trial. *Psychological Services, 15*(4), 386–397. doi: 10.1037/ser0000184

Kassinove, H., & Tafrate, R. C. (2002). *Anger management: The complete treatment guidebook for practitioners.* Oakland, CA: Impact Publishers.

Lewin, K. (1951). *Field theory in social science: Selected theoretical papers.* New York, NY: Harper & Brothers.

Maier, G. J., Stava, L. J., Morrow, B. R., van Rybroek, G. J., & Bauman, K. G. (1987). A model for understanding and managing cycles of aggression among psychiatric inpatients. *Hospital & Community Psychiatry, 38*(5), 520–524.

Maiuro, R. D. (1987). Gold award: Helping angry and violent people manage their emotions and behavior. *Hospital and Community Psychiatry, 38*(11), 1,207–1,210.

Morland, L. A., Greene, C. J., Rosen, C. S., Foy, D., Reilly, P., Shore, J., ... Frueh, B. C. (2010). Telemedicine for anger management therapy in a rural population of combat veterans with post-traumatic stress disorder: A randomized non-inferiority trial. *The Journal of Clinical Psychiatry, 71*(7), 855–863. doi: 10.4088/JCP.09m05604blu

Nolan, K. A., Czobor, P., Roy, B. B., Platt, M. M., Shope, C. B., Citrome, L. L., & Volavka, J. (2003). Characteristics of assaultive behavior among psychiatric inpatients. *Psychiatric Services, 54*(7), 1,012–1,016.

Petruzzello, S. J., Landers, D. M., Hatfield, B., Kubitz, K. A., & Salazar, W. (1991). A meta-analysis on the anxiety-reducing effects of acute and chronic exercise. Outcomes and mechanisms. *Sports Medicine, 11*(3), 141–182.

Schiraldi, G. R., & Kerr, M. H. (2002). *The anger management sourcebook.* New York, NY: McGraw-Hill Education.

Seaward, B. L. (2012). *Managing stress: Principles and strategies for health and well-being* (7th ed.). Burlington, VT: Jones & Bartlett Learning.

Shorey, R. C., McNulty, J. K., Moore, T. M., & Stuart, G. L. (2017). Trait anger and partner-specific anger management moderate the temporal association between alcohol use and dating violence. *Journal of Studies on Alcohol and Drugs, 78*(2), 313–318.

Shorey, R. C., Seavey, A. E., Quinn, E., & Cornelius, T. L. (2014). Partner-specific anger management as a mediator of the relation between mindfulness and female perpetrated dating violence. *Psychology of Violence, 4*(1), 51–64.

Tang, Y. Y., Hölzel, B. K., & Posner, M. I. (2015). The neuroscience of mindfulness meditation, *Nature Reviews Neuroscience, 16*(4), 213–225. doi: 10.1038/nrn3916

Walitzer, K. S., Deffenbacher, J. L., & Shyhalla, K. (2015). Alcohol-adapted anger management treatment: A randomized controlled trial of an innovative therapy for alcohol dependence. *Journal of Substance Abuse Treatment, 59*, 83–93. doi: 10.1016/j.jsat.2015.08.003

17

STAYING SAFE DURING DE-ESCALATION

"The care of human life and happiness, and not their destruction,
is the first and only object of good government."

–Thomas Jefferson

OBJECTIVES

- Study door safety protocols

- Grasp the importance of paying attention to your surroundings

- Find out how much space patients need

- Assess the effects of body language

- Find out what hairstyles and accessories pose a risk

- Evaluate the dangers of threatening patients

With any intervention, the goal is to obtain assistance as quickly as possible while at the same time preventing harm such as physical injury (Chabora, Judge-Gorny, & Grogan, 2003). That means keeping yourself, the patient, and everyone in the area safe and secure.

Of course, the entire de-escalation process is focused on safety—from intervening early, to knowing and using de-escalation techniques, to maintaining control of yourself and the situation, to ensuring positive communication, and so on. That's not what this chapter is about. Instead, this chapter discusses steps that you can take that relate *specifically* to safety to ensure the welfare of all involved. These include implementing certain safety protocols such as door safety protocols, paying attention to your surroundings, giving the patient plenty of room, watching your body language, avoiding clothing or accessories that might put you at risk, always having colleagues on hand to help, and more.

IMPLEMENT DOOR SAFETY PROTOCOLS

In mental health units, nurses are taught to stay close to the door in case they need to exit the area for safety reasons. This technique is useful for all healthcare nurses and staff.

Pay attention when a patient gets between you and the exit. If a patient who is agitated or aggressive, or exhibiting threatening behavior, positions himself between you and the door, it could mean you are in imminent physical danger. Were the patient to escalate to violence, you could be cornered or trapped—unable to get past the patient to escape. It's critical that nurses and other healthcare workers recognize this behavior as an indicator of danger in the healthcare environment (Stokowski, 2007).

On a related note, anytime you enter the room of a patient on an inpatient mental health unit, you must keep a clear path to the exit available. This may mean moving the patient's bedside table and any other obstacles out of the way. Position yourself so you have an easy unobstructed path to exit the room safely and quickly (Stokowski, 2007), and stay close to the door if you can.

> ✅ **NOTE** When in a patient's room, try to position yourself so the exit is accessible to both you *and* the patient. This may help reduce anxiety and tension for both of you.

PAY ATTENTION TO YOUR SURROUNDINGS

During any de-escalation scenario, you must pay attention to your surroundings (Berring, Pedersen, & Buus, 2016). Visually scan the perimeter. Look for objects that could be turned into weapons or projectiles. Make sure you have an unobstructed exit route. Finally, notice whether any coworkers are nearby in case you need help. (More on that later in this chapter.)

GIVE THE PATIENT ROOM

While conversing with agitated or aggressive patients, maintain a safe distance from them, and stay well outside their personal space (Gately & Stabb, 2005; Hilgers, 2003). (This is referred to as "proxemics.") For most people, their "personal space" consists of a 3- to 4-foot buffer. When patients are behaving in an aggressive manner, you should give them even more room. This ensures you will be beyond their reach and away from danger in the event they turn violent (Paterson, Leadbetter, & McComish, 1997). It also gives the patients room to breathe.

> **⚠ CAUTION** If a patient would be in a position to grab, hit, or kick you after taking just one step, then you are standing too close. Step back a few feet to give the patient space.

WATCH YOUR BODY LANGUAGE

Chapter 4, "De-Escalation Techniques," discussed the importance of watching your body language—your demeanor, facial expression, posture, gestures, and movement—to avoid upsetting patients unnecessarily. With respect to safety, it's important to take special care to avoid using body language that may be interpreted as intimidating or threatening. This helps ensure patients don't become violent in reaction to their fear that they are in danger. Here are a few specific tips:

- **Move slowly.** To avoid startling agitated patients, avoid sudden or abrupt movements, and approach them in clear view.

- **Maintain eye contact...** This shows your respect for the patients (Tingleff, Bradley, Gildberg, Munksgaard, & Hounsgaard, 2017).

- **...But not too much.** Some eye contact is good. But too much might be perceived as a challenge or threat.

- **Speak at eye level.** This conveys that you see the patients as equals. If necessary, sit down next to them to achieve this.

- **Don't stand over the patients.** This makes the patients feel as though you are looking down on them. Always speak to patients at their eye level.

- **Don't back patients into a corner.** Being backed into a corner can intensify patients' anxiety and paranoia, leading to agitation and panic. When patients are cornered, they fight. Give them space and an exit route to prevent them from feeling trapped.

- **Don't crowd patients.** Give patients plenty of space. Put at least 3 to 4 feet of distance between yourself and them during de-escalation. If patients have a history of aggression or violence, give them even more room. This will decrease their anxiety (as well as your own) and enable successful de-escalation.

- **Don't touch the patients.** This could be interpreted as an aggressive gesture (Paterson et al., 1997).

- **Don't turn your back on the patients.** This prevents you from monitoring the patients visually and places you in a vulnerable position.

- **Keep your hands free and in the open.** Some patients feel threatened if they cannot see your hands. As an added bonus, keeping your hands free and in the open means you will be better able to quickly defend yourself if patients attack.

- **Don't cross your arms.** Crossing your arms conveys a harsh and hostile message to patients (Mohr, 2009).

- **Adopt a supportive stance.** In this stance, the feet are shoulder width apart, the arms are bent slightly, and the hands are open in front of the thighs with the palms facing upward (Hallett & Dickens, 2017). (See Figure 17.1.) This stance is a nonverbal way to convey that you are not a threat. It communicates kindness, courtesy, and respect (National Health Service, 2008). This stands in contrast to a fighting stance, which will generally be interpreted as menacing—especially if you are standing right in front of patients.

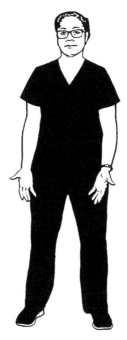

FIGURE 17.1 Adopt a supportive stance.

BE MINDFUL OF HAIR AND ACCESSORIES

If you have long hair, avoid wearing it loose. An aggressive patient could easily injure you by pulling it or tangling fingers into it to hold you in place (Stokowski, 2007). Hair is safest when worn short or in a bun.

Dangle earrings are also a danger. As with hair, a patient could grab and pull dangle earrings. Or, the earrings could be pulled accidentally by a coworker during a therapeutic containment (takedown) event. If earrings must be worn, post earrings without dangles are best. Neck jewelry is also best avoided due to the risk for strangulation. Heavy neck chains are particularly dangerous. For your safety, it's best to leave this type of jewelry at home.

In addition to neck jewelry, badge cords and stethoscopes worn around the neck pose a risk for strangulation. Fortunately, most hospitals provide nurses with breakaway lanyard badge cords for safety reasons. As for stethoscopes, it's best to carry yours in your hand or pocket rather than wearing it around your neck.

> **⚠ CAUTION** Remove dangerous objects from your person. Discard any pens, sharp objects, or cords before approaching a patient to de-escalate.

DON'T THREATEN THE PATIENT

Nurses sometimes threaten patients in a healthcare environment inadvertently. For example, they might tell a patient that they'll have to administer an injection or use a restraint if the patient doesn't stop acting out (Dickinson, Ramsdale, & Speight, 2009). This is a mistake. Threats will only intensify the patient's anger or fear and often result in violence (Haggård-Grann, Hallqvist, Långström, & Möller, 2006; Lanza, Kayne, Hicks, & Milner, 1991). On a related note, avoid arguing with the patient or being confrontational. This could cause the patient's behavior to escalate.

> **⚠ CAUTION** Simply put, threats have no place in a healthcare environment. It's far better to collaborate with the patient to de-escalate the situation. Remember: Collaborate, don't intimidate!

KEEP A COWORKER NEARBY

Although it's wise to remove the patient from an audience of peers, you should never be alone with an agitated or aggressive person. For safety reasons, have a coworker stand by, or ask a security guard for assistance.

When faced with an aggressive patient, use the "buddy system." Know where your coworkers are, and watch out for each other. It's a good practice to develop silent hand signals to summon help from your "buddy" when faced with an aggressive patient. For example, you might hold up two fingers in the "peace" or "victory" sign. This serves as a signal to nearby staff that you need help.

If you suspect a patient will become aggressive or violent, summon help. It's better to have assistance available and not need it than to need assistance and not have it available. Call for help the instant you think you might need it. If a situation escalates to the point where the staff is afraid the patient might become violent—or the patient actually *does* become violent—notify security or police for safety.

Many mental health facilities and even some medical healthcare facilities provide behavioral emergency response teams—sometimes called crisis intervention teams (CITs)—to assist with de-escalation. These teams consist of highly trained healthcare professions who are skilled in crisis prevention intervention (CPI), safety, and de-escalation. The behavioral emergency response team responds to every behavioral code. The mental health nurse manager also responds, along with a therapist and security. Essentially, everyone trained in emergency behavioral response intervention arrives with the team.

One way to summon help from a behavioral emergency response team is to issue an overhead page with a designated code word or phrase, such as "Dr. Strong 4 North." Another method is to use a GPS-enabled panic button. These are often used in mental health units. Staff carry these devices and press them when in danger to issue a behavioral code that includes their location.

> ⚠ **CAUTION** No staff member should ever be left alone on an inpatient unit where they could be easily overpowered. You should always have at least two staff members on duty (Stokowski, 2007).

Other General Safety Tips

Here are some additional safety tips to ensure everyone remains safe during a de-escalation, or to help prevent an aggressive episode in the first place:

- **Design the ward for optimal observation.** The best ward design is one in which staff have an unobstructed view of patients in communal areas such as dayrooms, dining rooms, and hallways. Ideally, curved Plexiglas mirrors will be placed at hallway intersections or concealed areas to maintain safety and visibility. Many facilities have also installed closed-circuit video recording cameras in high-risk areas. The feed from these cameras appears on a dashboard viewscreen at the nurses station.

- **Mitigate risks during times of transition.** Staff should be available for therapeutic intervention and de-escalation even during shift changes (Hamrin, Iennaco, & Olsen, 2009).

- **Stagger shifts so they overlap.** This prevents gaps in care during shift changes.

- **Conduct safety searches for hazardous items as per facility policy (mental health inpatient facilities only).** All patients admitted on an inpatient basis to a mental health facility are subjected to a hazardous item (contraband) safety search as per the facility protocol to remove any items that could pose a danger, such as glass, metal, and cords

continues

(ligatures). Some mental health facilities have also begun implementing metal detector scans to identify guns, knives, or other weapons—not just for patients, but for every person who enters the mental health unit—to ensure a safe environment for everyone.

- **Control access to entrances and exits.** As a safety intervention, medical facilities lock unused doors to limit access in accordance with local fire codes. This eliminates the danger of outsiders entering the facility at night to possibly cause harm. Controlled access to patient areas reduces the risk of physical assault (Gillespie, Gates, Miller, & Howard, 2010).

CASE STUDY

USING THE "BUDDY SYSTEM"

Mr. Lewis is a 53-year-old man with an acquired brain injury from a motor vehicle accident. Since undergoing an operation to replace his right hip a month ago, he has developed an unsteady gait. Current diagnoses are psychotic disorder NOS and concussive dementia. Mr. Lewis presents as being irritable, labile, demanding, and confused. Mr. Lewis requires assistance with all activities of daily living (ADLs), including toileting, dressing, nutrition, and ambulation.

The nurse on duty, Samantha, hears Mr. Lewis shouting in his room that he needs a nurse to take him to the bathroom. She immediately walks into his room. When she does, she sees Mr. Lewis attempting to get out of bed without assistance. Mr. Lewis then begins waving his arms wildly and cursing Samantha. Samantha recognizes that Mr. Lewis is agitated and requires immediate de-escalation.

Samantha activates the "buddy system" by asking a second nurse, Oliver, to stand watch. Oliver stands calmly in the doorway. He does not speak to or touch Mr. Lewis as Samantha gently redirects him. This prevents Mr. Lewis from being overwhelmed by too much communication. Samantha begins speaking to Mr. Lewis in a slow, calm, and direct manner, while standing outside his personal space. As she does, Oliver continues to stand quietly in the doorway, ready to assist Samantha if needed for safety.

Samantha continues to speak to Mr. Lewis in a calm and pleasant manner. She asks his permission to assist him and explains that she will gladly help him to the bathroom. Mr. Lewis agrees to walk to the bathroom with her assistance and begins to calm down. After he is finished in the bathroom, Samantha helps Mr. Lewis back into bed. Finally, Samantha suggests to Mr. Lewis that he rest for a while in the quiet of his room. Through it all, Oliver stands quietly in the doorway, poised to help.

Later, Samantha returns to Mr. Lewis's room. She sits down with him to discuss his earlier anger. During the conversation, Mr. Lewis explains that his anger arose because he thought he would not be able to get to the bathroom in time. He then states that all he needs is for someone to come by every so often to help him go to the bathroom, and he will not become so angry again. Samantha agrees to place Mr. Lewis on a two-hour toileting schedule and informs the healthcare team of the change for continuity of care.

With early intervention with de-escalation, and therapeutic communication skills, Samantha has found a way to prevent future episodes with Mr. Lewis and improve unit safety.

REFERENCES

Berring, L. L., Pedersen, L., & Buus, N. (2016). Coping with violence in mental health care settings: Patient and staff member perspectives on de-escalation practices. *Archives of Psychiatric Nursing, 30*(5), 499–507. doi: 10.1016/j.apnu.2016.05.005

Chabora, N., Judge-Gorny, M., & Grogan, K. (2003). The Four S Model in Action for de-escalation: An innovative state hospital-university collaborative endeavor. *Journal of Psychosocial Nursing and Mental Health Services, 41*(1), 22–28.

Dickinson, T., Ramsdale, S., & Speight, G. (2009). Managing aggression and violence using rapid tranquillisation. *Nursing Standard, 24*(7), 40–49.

Gately, L. A., & Stabb, S. D. (2005). Psychology students' training in the management of potentially violent clients. *Professional Psychology: Research and Practice, 36*(6), 681–687.

Gillespie, G. L., Gates, D. M., Miller, M., & Howard, P. K. (2010). Workplace violence in healthcare settings: Risk factors and protective strategies. *Rehabilitation Nursing, 35*(5), 177–184.

Haggård-Grann, U., Hallqvist, J., Långström, N., & Möller, J. (2006). Short-term effects of psychiatric symptoms and interpersonal stressors on criminal violence: A case-crossover study. *Social Psychiatry and Psychiatric Epidemiology, 41*(7), 532–540.

Hallett, N., & Dickens, G. L. (2017). De-escalation of aggressive behavior in healthcare settings: Concept analysis. *International Journal of Nursing Studies, 75*, 10–20. doi: 10.1016/j.ijnurstu.2017.07.003

Hamrin, V., Iennaco, J., & Olsen, D. (2009). A review of ecological factors affecting inpatient psychiatric unit violence: Implications for relational and unit cultural improvements. *Issues in Mental Health Nursing, 30*(4), 214–226. doi: 10.1080/01612840802701083

Hilgers, J. (2003). Comforting a confused patient. *Nursing, 33*(1), 48–50.

Lanza, M. L., Kayne, H. L., Hicks, C., & Milner, J. (1991). Nursing staff characteristics related to patient assault. *Issues in Mental Health Nursing, 12*(3), 253–265.

Mohr, W. K. (2009). *Psychiatric-mental health nursing: Evidenced-based concepts, skills, and practices* (7th ed.). Philadelphia, PA: Lippincott Williams & Wilkins.

National Health Service. (2008). *Policy and guidance for the recognition, prevention and therapeutic management of violence and aggression.* North East London Foundation Trust.

Paterson, B., Leadbetter, D., & McComish, A. (1997). De-escalation in the management of aggression and violence. *Nursing Times, 93*(36), 58–61.

Stokowski, L. (2007). Alternatives to restraint and seclusion in mental health settings: Questions and answers from psychiatric nurse experts. *Medscape*. Retrieved from https://www.medscape.com/viewarticle/555686

Tingleff, E. B., Bradley, S. K., Gildberg, F. A., Munksgaard, G., & Hounsgaard, L. (2017). "Treat me with respect." A systematic review and thematic analysis of psychiatric patients' reported perceptions of the situations associated with the process of coercion. *Journal of Psychiatric and Mental Health Nursing, 24*(9), 681–698. doi: 10.1111/jpm.12410

18

AFTER THE INCIDENT

"We are all invited to work together for peace. We shall join hands and minds to work for peace through active nonviolence. We shall help one another, encourage one another and learn from one another how to bring peace to our children and to all."

–Mairead Corrigan Maguire

OBJECTIVES

- Cover debriefing after an aggressive episode
- Find out how to report and document a de-escalation encounter

After any de-escalation event, when things have calmed down, it's important to conduct a debrief with both the patient and other staff, and to report and document the incident. This helps reduce the chances of it being repeated.

DEBRIEFING WITH THE PATIENT AND STAFF

Debriefing is defined as an official questioning session after an event—an interview in which the patient, nurse, and any other staff present for the de-escalation event are asked about and asked to report on the incident. The process of the debriefing is documented and becomes part of the electronic health record.

Debriefing is not a choice. Debriefing is a Joint Commission (JC) mandated process for all mental health facilities (2019). The JC requires every facility to have written policies and procedures for debriefing. In best practice applications, mental health facilities debrief after every behavioral emergency code (silent or called). Debriefs are also completed after every assault. Finally, debriefs are required after every use of four-point behavioral restraints (on all four extremities)—whether in a mental health facility or a medical facility (including the emergency department). Debriefings must occur within a specific timeframe. The JC allows 24 hours to complete a debriefing. The JC reviews debriefing documentation during annual surveys for accuracy and completion.

A debriefing session is a powerful opportunity for everyone involved in a crisis—including the patient—to examine and share feelings and perceptions about the incident. Patients and staff alike are encouraged to speak about what occurred and to talk about how they feel about what happened. Reviewing the traumatic experience in this way allows those involved to process it and helps to mitigate any damage that might result from the event (Kaplan, Iancu, & Bodner, 2001). Debriefings also offer an opportunity to review clinical data, revise the patient's treatment plan, and identify opportunities for performance improvement.

> ☑ **NOTE** The inclusion of the patient's perspective in any debriefing is critical.

Debriefing is a teaching moment. It demonstrates how to work with individuals who are engaging in inappropriate behaviors to help them identify what those behaviors are and to problem-solve and identify how to do something better and differently. The goal of any debriefing is to prevent problems rather than place blame. The debriefing should focus on addressing what can be learned from the incident and how staff and patients can use that knowledge to prevent it from happening again. It provides an opportunity to review techniques used and to consider lessons learned. Debriefing is about identifying what can be changed to avoid an aggressive episode in the future.

> ✅ **NOTE** Debriefings often reveal interventions that could help prevent future acts of aggression or violence.

The clinical impact of the intervention on the patient should also be reviewed (American Psychiatric Association (APA), American Academy of Child & Adolescent Psychiatry (AACAP), & National Association of Psychiatric Health Systems (NAPHS), 1999). During debriefing, the patient should be asked about feelings at the time of the episode and a description of any precipitating events that led to the agitation. Some patients might refuse to discuss details of the incident at first. With gentle therapeutic encouragement, however, these patients may soften and begin to talk about what happened.

Typically, the person assigned to conduct the debriefing is a designated charge nurse, nurse manager, supervisor, or house supervisor (during after-hours). This person should direct the following questions to everyone involved in the incident and record each person's replies using an electronic template:

- Who was involved?

- What happened?

- Where did it happen?

- What caused it to happen?

- How can we prevent it from happening again?

> ✅ **NOTE** It is important to consider and incorporate the way that all involved persons—including members of the patient community, when appropriate—can be included in the debriefing (APA, AACAP, & NAPHS, 1999).

Joint Commission Requirements for Debriefing

Following are the JC requirements for debriefings:

1. The patient and, if appropriate, the patient's family should participate in a debriefing with available staff members who were involved in each episode involving the use of restraint or seclusion.

2. The debriefing should occur as soon as possible and appropriate, but no longer than 24 hours after the episode.

3. The debriefing is used to do the following:

   - Identify what led to the incident and what could have been handled differently.

   - Ascertain that the patient's physical well-being, psychological comfort, and right to privacy were addressed.

   - Counsel the patient for any trauma that may have resulted from the incident.

   - When indicated, modify the patient's plan for care, treatment, and services.

4. Information obtained and documented from debriefings should be used in performance-improvement activities.

(JC, 2019)

REPORTING AND DOCUMENTING A DE-ESCALATION ENCOUNTER

Healthcare staff must report de-escalation encounters to the provider on duty, such as a physician, psychiatrist, or nurse practitioner. The nurse manager or supervisor on duty should also be notified. In addition, information about the intervention should be included in the unit report to inform nurses arriving on duty. Finally, some facilities may require the completion of an incident report.

Staff must also document the de-escalation encounter. This documentation should include the following:

- The date and time of the de-escalation encounter

- An objective description of the patient's behavior and verbalizations, using quotes if possible

- The specific de-escalation techniques used, and any other care provided to the patient during the encounter

- The patient's response to these interactions

- A description of your contacts with the patient during the incident, step by step

- The names and times of persons notified of the patient's behavior and their response (Mohr, 2009)—for example, the attending physician or the psychiatrist on duty

- What time the notified individuals arrived to see the patient

- Whether the de-escalation intervention was successful

This information will be communicated to all members of the healthcare team for future reference.

It is vital to accurately document de-escalation. This verifies the use of best practice, least-restrictive de-escalation interventions. The JC requires the use of least-restrictive interventions such as de-escalation during behavioral episodes. Only facilities with low use of PRN (when needed) medication, restraint, and seclusion, and high use of de-escalation techniques, meet the JC's high standards of quality care.

During surveys, the JC audits patient charts to determine if de-escalation techniques were attempted and documented prior to the use of PRN medications such as lorazepam or haloperidol. If there is no documentation of an attempt to de-escalate before using a PRN medication, restraints, or seclusion, the facility may be marked as substandard in care. Therefore, every de-escalation event must be reported and documented (Snorrason & Biering, 2018).

> ✅ **NOTE** Medical and mental health facilities' electronic health record documentation templates feature clinical pop-up reminder boxes to prompt you to document de-escalation attempts made prior to use of PRN medication. This is required by all medical and mental health facilities.

Therapeutic Interdisciplinary Team Communication

Communication among interdisciplinary healthcare personnel is very important for providing therapeutic, patient-centered care. This allows for consistency in care and early intervention with de-escalation techniques.

Reporting and documentation are essential forms of interdisciplinary communication. When staff observe that a particular de-escalation technique is effective in calming a patient, this information should be placed in a report to inform other members of the healthcare team so they can use the same technique if needed.

It is vital that all interdisciplinary communication be accurate, clear, concise, and consistent. Clear interdisciplinary communication is essential for quality care and improved patient outcomes (Grover, 2005).

REFERENCES

American Psychiatric Association, American Academy of Child & Adolescent Psychiatry, & National Association of Psychiatric Health Systems. (1999). *Joint statement of general principles on seclusion and restraint.*

Grover, S. (2005). Shaping effective communication skills and therapeutic relationships at work: The foundation of communication. *AAOHN Journal, 53*(4), 177–182.

The Joint Commission. (2019). *2019 comprehensive accreditation manual for hospitals.* Oak Brook, IL: Joint Commission.

Kaplan, Z., Iancu, I., & Bodner, E. (2001). A review of psychological debriefing after extreme stress. *Psychiatric Services, 52*(6), 824–827.

Mohr, W. K. (2009). *Psychiatric-mental health nursing: Evidenced-based concepts, skills, and practices* (7th ed.). Philadelphia, PA: Lippincott Williams & Wilkins.

Snorrason, J., & Biering, P. (2018). The attributes of successful de-escalation and restraint teams. *International Journal of Mental Health Nursing, 27*(6), 1,842–1,850. doi: 10.1111/inm.12493

CREATING A CALMING, CARING, AND HEALING HEALTHCARE ENVIRONMENT

"Education breeds confidence, confidence breeds hope, hope breeds peace."

–Confucius

OBJECTIVES

- Discuss how to create a caring and healing physical environment

- Find out how to foster a caring and healing environment through staff interactions

- Examine an effective caring model

- Explore caring theory

In any clinical setting, the healthcare environment can either create or mitigate stress. A healthcare environment that is caring and healing does the latter—decreasing stress and creating a supportive space for healing by inducing calm and serenity and inhibiting agitation and aggression (Sakallaris, MacAllister, Voss, Smith, & Jonas, 2015).

Medical facilities have discovered the benefits of a caring and healing environment to promote physical healing as well as mental health. Indeed, research shows that a caring-healing environment has a positive impact in both physical and psychological recovery outcomes (Gouin, Kiecolt-Glaser, Malarkey, & Glaser, 2007).

The healthcare environment includes the physical layout and design of a patient's room, hallways, and unit, and the facility as a whole. But it also includes the staff (Keegan, 1994; Kreitzer, 2015). That is, the healthcare environment isn't just about the facility; it's about every interaction between staff and patients *inside* the facility. Indeed, these interactions play the biggest role in fostering a caring-healing environment. Although the physical healthcare environment enhances healing, it is the spirit and presence of the healthcare staff that is most vital.

It's not just nurses who contribute to a caring-healing environment. Every member of the healthcare team who interacts with a patient plays a role, including doctors, admission clerks, transport staff, dietary staff, housekeeping staff, administrative staff, and the business office staff (Foss Durant, McDermott, Kinney, & Triner, 2015). Environments that are truly healing and caring are created when interpersonal relationships between caregivers and those they serve are built on mutual respect and a shared commitment to holistic healing (Felgen, 2003).

CREATING A CARING AND HEALING PHYSICAL ENVIRONMENT

Nature themes are a key element of caring-healing environments. Environments with views of or access to nature areas such as gardens and fountains are shown to improve cohesion of mind, body, and spirit (Sakallaris et al., 2015). Indeed, research by Ulrich (1984) demonstrated that placing post-surgery patients in a room with a window overlooking a pleasant nature scene resulted in shorter hospital stays and improved attitudes, mood, and behavior. Patients in these rooms also required fewer prescribed analgesics than those without a view. In areas without access to or views of nature, nature-based artwork can help create a calming and restorative space. So too can calming messages—for example, posters with words like "Peace" and "Hope."

> ✅ **NOTE** Patients consider a healthcare environment to be "healing" when they have positive relationships with caregivers; when care attends to the body, emotions, mind, and spirit; when they have a relationship with their caregiver; and when they are actively involved in decisions regarding their own care.

FOSTERING CARING AND HEALING HEALTHCARE ENVIRONMENTS THROUGH STAFF INTERACTIONS

An intentional caring relationship between a caregiver and patient (and the family) is the core of the healing environment. This requires compassion and empathy. *Compassion* refers to an awareness and understanding of one's relationship to all living beings. *Empathy* is the ability to step into another's shoes.

Caring presence is another requirement. Caring presence is not just "being there" in a physical sense. It's paying attention to, being profoundly present for, and showing caring for patients in every interaction—even while attending to routine or repetitive tasks. A caring presence is the foundation of the therapeutic nurse-patient relationship and the cornerstone of a caring-healing environment. It's what enables healthcare staff to establish trust and rapport with patients and family members (Felgen, 2004; Keegan, 1994; Trout, 2011). A caring presence can also help prevent escalation and assist with de-escalation.

> ✅ **NOTE** Healing relationships require therapeutic communication, emotional self-management, and the ability to be truly present in each encounter to offer unconditional caring (Douglas, Hathaway, & Burks, 2011; Sakallaris et al., 2015).

Caring is most often expressed in what are called "moments of caring." Moments of caring occur in the interpersonal interactions between staff and patients, families, visitors, or colleagues (Felgen, 2004). These shared moments can make the difference in a patient's opinion of the healthcare staff and the facility as a whole and can leave a positive impact for the rest of the patient's life. Even the simple act of helping a patient eat or teaching a family member to provide essential care at home are moments of caring. Other examples of caring moments that create a sacred space to heal and calm include:

- An admission clerk efficiently completing the patient's paperwork with kindness and respect

- A nurse patiently answering a patient's many questions and listening to the patient's concerns with caring and compassion

- A member of the transport staff stopping to kindly redirect a visitor who is lost

- A member of the housekeeping smiling while working to clean the patient's room

In addition, the administrative staff creates a caring and healing environment when they advocate for patient and human rights, and the business office staff creates a caring and healing environment when they keep the patient's accounts accurately and responsibly.

Building Collegial Relationships to Foster a Caring and Healing Environment

It's impossible to foster a caring and healing environment if staff morale is low. Staff morale has a direct impact on patient care.

A key driver of staff morale is the existence of collegial relationships among members of interdisciplinary teams. Indeed, collegial interdisciplinary relationships are *the* foundation of effective working groups (Saltus, 2011).

Collegial relationships are characterized by four key qualities: trust; mutual respect; support; and open, honest communication. When these qualities are present, team members recognize each other as colleagues, driving positive interactions and collaboration (Koloroutis, 2004; Sakallaris et al., 2015).

Developing collegial interdisciplinary relationships takes time, commitment, dedication, and energy, but it's worth it.

> ✓ **NOTE** Every patient encounter is an opportunity to show someone you care, and every act of kindness is a moment of caring.

A MODEL FOR CARING BEHAVIOR

Establishing a caring model helps to foster a caring and healing healthcare environment. A caring model consists of three key components (Schwerin, 2004):

- **Care of the self.** Nurses cannot care for others until they have nurtured themselves.

- **Care of each other.** As nurses, we must always display kindness toward each other. Be good to your coworkers. Life is difficult enough *without* the stressors that accompany interpersonal conflicts.

- **Care for patients.** We are privileged to serve our patients.

Sharing kindness with each other in a healthcare environment represents a "moment of caring" that can make this world a better place for everyone.

> ✅ **NOTE** A caring and healing environment is one that carefully attends to the entire experience of patients and families and acknowledges and values its practitioners (Jarrin, 2012; Keegan, 1994).

CARING THEORY

Nursing theorists have developed various theories that pertain to the concept of human caring to create a vibrant healthcare environment that promotes optimal healing and recovery.

One of these theories is the Model of Human Care by theorist Jean Watson. Watson's model points to the significance of a caring-healing consciousness in transforming the patient's healthcare experience into a positive caring experience and posits that the whole caring-healing consciousness is contained within a single caring moment (Watson, 2002).

Watson's model outlines three key concepts (Watson & Foster, 2003):

- **Only the patient can change herself.** A person cannot be forced into change. Attempting this may cause agitation. The person must want to change from within, or you will never be able to facilitate change. The nurse's duty is to promote helpful, calming, healing change, while supporting the patient's dignity and recovery from illness or injury.

■ **Healing comes from the inside out.** The will to heal comes from within. A nurse's duty in the patient's illness experience is to provide for the patient holistic, healing, calming care. The nurse's commitment to caring is to alleviate pain, stress, and suffering. The nurse as a caring professional promotes the well-being, healing, and harmony of the mind, body, and spirit of the one being cared for.

■ **The nurse facilitates healing changes.** Nurses facilitate healing through compassionate practice. In caring moments, nurses provide holistic care, nurturing the healing process. They assist with basic needs and attend to the unity of being in the caring consciousness, promoting calming, healing, and recovery from the experience of illness and trauma.

Watson's theory also describes several crucial principles:

■ **The one caring and the one being cared for are interconnected.** The nurse and the patient must act as partners in recovery-oriented care. Nurses facilitate best practices in nursing care by articulating calming and caring behaviors to help build trusting relationships. Nurses connect in the caring-healing relationship with patients in daily care, nurturing holistic recovery of the mind, body, and spirit.

■ **The human caring and healing processes are communicated to the one being cared for.** Caring and healing processes are communicated by healing pathways of recovery-oriented care. Nurses are accepting of patients not only as they are but also as what they may become. Respect is nurtured in the relationship as the patients are understood, assisted, and valued in their everyday existence.

■ **Caring and healing consciousness is extended through space and time.** The caring-healing relationship exists in every act of human caring and is sustained through space and time in the science of human caring. The intentional caring consciousness exists in each and every moment of imparted caring. Nurses administer care to all aspects of the patient's mind-body experience, evolving into spiritual growth and self-actualization.

■ **Caring-healing consciousness is dominant over physical illness and treatment.** The practice of caring is the center of all holistic, recovery-oriented nursing care. Effective care in the nurse-patient relationship promotes health and growth for the patient and the patient's family. Creative use of self in the healing process empowers caring and healing environments, whereby wholeness, beauty, peace, and comfort are made possible for holistic healing.

Another caring theory is the Culture Care Diversity and Universality Theory by theorist Madeline Leininger (2006). This theory expresses five theoretical assumptions about caring (Leininger, 2006):

- Care is essential for human growth and survival, and eventually to face death.

- There cannot be curing without caring.

- Expressions of human care vary among all world cultures.

- Therapeutic nursing care can only occur when cultural care values, expressions, and practices are known and used.

- Nursing is a transcultural care profession and discipline.

These caring assumptions form the basis of *universal culture caring*, which is the fundamental right to holistic human caring that transcends all communities, cultures, and nationalities. According to Leininger (2006), several universal caring characteristics are common to all cultures on Earth:

- Respect

- Concern for self and other

- Helping, assisting, and facilitating

- Paying attention to details

- Presence

- Connecting

- Protecting

- Touching

- Comfort

- Environmental accommodation to provide comfort

> ✅ **NOTE** Respect is an essential characteristic of human caring. When we show respect for others, we teach them to respect themselves; when they respect themselves, they can learn to respect others.

REFERENCES

Douglas, K., Hathaway, R., & Burks, S. (2011). 'The environment matters' and 'designing toward the whole.' *Nursing Economic$, 29*(1), 42–45.

Felgen, J. A. (2003). Caring core value, currency, and commodity…is it time to get tough about "soft"? *Nursing Administrator Quarterly, 27*(3), 208–214. doi: 10.1097/00006216-200307000-00007

Felgen, J. A. (2004). A caring and healing environment. *Nursing Administration Quarterly, 28*(4), 288–301. doi: 10.1097/00006216-200410000-00012

Foss Durant, A., McDermott, S., Kinney, G., & Triner, T. (2015). Caring science: Transforming the ethic of caring-healing practice, environment, and culture within an integrated care delivery system. *Permanente Journal, 19*(4), 136–142.

Gouin, J. P., Kiecolt-Glaser, J. K., Malarkey, W. B., & Glaser, R. (2007). The influence of anger expression on wound healing. *Brain, Behavior, and Immunity, 22*(5), 699–708.

Jarrin, O. F. (2012). The integrality of situated caring in nursing and the environment. *Advances in Nursing Science, 35*(1), 14–24. doi: 10.1097/ANS.0b013c3182433b89

Keegan, L. (1994). *The nurse as healer.* Albany, NY: Delmar Publishers.

Koloroutis, M. (2004). *Relationship-based care: A model for transforming practice.* Minneapolis, MN: Creative Health Care Management, Inc.

Kreitzer, M. J. (2015). Integrative nursing: Application of principles across clinical settings. *Rambam Maimonides Medical Journal, 6*(2), e0016. doi: 10.5041/RMMJ.10200

Leininger, M. M. (2006). *Culture care diversity and universality: A worldwide nursing theory* (2nd ed.). Burlington, MA: Jones & Bartlett Learning.

Sakallaris, B. R., MacAllister, L., Voss, M., Smith, K., & Jonas, W. B. (2015). Optimal healing environments. *Global Advances in Health Medicine, 4*(3), 40–45. doi: 10.7453/gahmj.2015.043

Saltus, G. L. (2011). Who am I in this work? *Creative Nursing, 17*(1), 22–24.

Schwerin, J. I. (2004). The timeless caring connection. *Nursing Administration Quarterly, 28*(4), 265–270.

Trout, M. (2011). Presence and attunement in health care: A view from infancy research. *Creative Nursing, 17*(1), 16–21.

Ulrich, R. S. (1984). View through a window may influence recovery from surgery. *Science, 224*(4647), 420–421.

Watson, J. (2002). Intentionality and caring-healing consciousness: A practice of transpersonal nursing. *Holistic Nursing Practice, 16*(4), 12–19.

Watson, J., & Foster, R. (2003). The attending nurse caring model: Integrating theory, evidence, and advanced caring-healing therapeutics for transforming professional practice. *Journal of Clinical Nursing, 12*(3), 360–365.

DEVELOPING A HEALTHCARE VIOLENCE-PREVENTION PLAN

"It isn't enough to talk about peace. One must believe in it. And it isn't enough to believe in it. One must work at it."

–Eleanor Roosevelt

OBJECTIVES

- Outline patient risk factors and effective interventions

- Specify environmental risk factors and effective interventions

- Delineate caregiver risk factors and effective interventions

- Find out how to put all this information together into a healthcare violence-prevention plan

To prevent violence in the healthcare setting, you need a plan. This plan must account for common causes of violence, include specific techniques to prevent violence, and cite interventional strategies to de-escalate violent situations when they occur. Assembling a plan and a de-escalation educational program to combat violence in a healthcare setting helps foster a therapeutic environment and promotes safety, health, wellness, and optimal recovery outcomes.

Essentially, this entire book is focused on developing your de-escalation plan and educational program to prevent violence. In Chapter 2, "Variables and Risk Factors for Aggression," you learned about common causes of violence, including patient variables, environmental variables, caregiver variables, and patient and caregiver interaction variables. Various chapters discussed specific techniques for preventing and de-escalating violence. And several chapters covered which techniques to use to de-escalate specific types of violent situations when they occur. This chapter simply helps you step through the process of actually assembling all this information to put your violence-prevention plan and de-escalation educational program into place. Organizing a healthcare violence-prevention plan by the holistic risk factor domains of patient, environment, and caregiver is an effective approach to preventing healthcare violence.

> ☑ **NOTE** As discussed throughout the book (but especially in Chapter 3, "Assessing an Escalating Situation for Early Intervention"), no matter what is causing a patient to escalate to behavior that is agitated, aggressive, or violent, early intervention is key—*before* the patient loses complete control. This breaks the cycle of aggression and prevents violence (Hodgins, 2008).

ADDRESSING PATIENT FACTORS

To review, patient factors indicating increased risk of aggression include the following:

- Mental instability

- The presence of delusions

- The presence of command hallucinations with violent content

- History of violence

- Poor impulse control

- Irritability

- Attention-seeking behavior

- An agitated state

- Disorganized thought processes

- Violation of personal space

Specific steps you can take to address these factors, and which should be delineated in your violence-prevention plan, include the following:

- **Perform mental status and risk assessment as per facility policy on admission.** This helps the provider identify triggers for aggression and factors that might help mitigate the risk of aggression—especially with early intervention. (Refer to Chapter 10, "Performing a Mental Status Assessment," for more information.)

- **Intervene and de-escalate early.** The earlier the intervention, the more likely it is to be successful.

- **Provide patient education.** The idea is to help patients develop coping skills and learn effective approaches for dealing with life's tough situations. Mental health facilities provide diverse group therapy education resources for inpatients. (Some of these groups are also available on an outpatient basis with provider referral.) These include the following:

  - Groups for people recovering from alcohol or substance abuse or addiction

  - Psycho-education groups to provide education on life skills and managing mental illness

  - Activity therapy groups in which patients engage in arts and crafts or music therapy

  - Cognitive behavioral therapy groups in which patients learn healthier ways of dealing with issues

  - Anger-management groups, to gain skills for coping with dysfunctional anger

  - Conflict-resolution groups, to educate patients on techniques to resolve psychosocial conflicts

  - Community groups, in which inpatients discuss and work through issues concerning their inpatient communities

- Groups for patients with certain symptoms, in which patients learn techniques to cope with pervasive symptoms of mental illness

- Groups for patients who take certain medications, in which patients learn about the uses and side effects of the medication

- Stress-management groups, in which patients learn techniques to relieve overwhelming stress

■ **Provide peer mentors for patient support.** Peer mentors are mental health patients in recovery from mental illness who are stable and volunteer to serve as a positive role model for change and recovery from mental illness.

■ **Provide patients with other outlets for stress and anxiety.** This could include physical exercise, listening to music, talking to a friend or staff member, attending a support group, and so on. Providing alternative means of channeling aggression and anger can help decrease anxiety and stress and promote calming.

■ **Allow for direct communication with caregivers and providers.** Open up lines of communication between the patient, provider, and interdisciplinary staff. Keeping communication lines open facilitates support and freedom of expression with regard to complex care issues and family dynamics. Open communication can also help resolve misunderstandings before they complicate care or grow into larger problems such as behavioral issues (American Psychiatric Association, American Psychiatric Nurses Association, & National Association of Psychiatric Health Systems, 2007).

■ **Collaborate with patients in treatment planning.** Personalize the treatment plan to focus on the patient's individual healthcare needs. Partner with the patient to identify and meet pertinent healthcare needs prior to discharge—for example, whether the patient will require a walker and need training on how to use it—and when continuing will follow-up home care. A patient whose healthcare needs are met is less likely to escalate from tension and stress than one whose needs go unmet.

■ **Emphasize patients' strengths and the hope of recovery.** Making patients aware of their strengths—such as a supportive family and a good prognosis—promotes hope for a holistic recovery. This reduces the risks of depression, despondency, and potential escalation to self-harming behaviors.

- **Identify incentives for optimal improvement.** Remind patients of incentives for recovery. For example, when caring for stroke patients, you could remind them of the incentive of returning home to encourage them to practice walking and to building up enough strength to walk on their own. You can use a similar incentive (or offer other privileges) for patients in a mental health facility to encourage them to improve behavioral control. Incentives gives patients a goal to reach for as they endeavor to meet the challenges of hospitalization and illness recovery.

- **Practice one-to-one observation (if called for).** De-escalation is a primary intervention for safety. For patients who pose a high risk for violence, close observation (one-to-one) may be ordered and implemented as a therapeutic safety intervention, with continuous monitoring as well as continuous de-escalation to prevent harm to self or others.

ADDRESSING ENVIRONMENTAL FACTORS

As discussed, environmental factors that may increase the risk of aggression include:

- Excessive motion

- Excessive noxious noise

- Lack of stimulation

- The ever-changing inpatient population

- The unpredictable behavior of others

- Crowded inpatient facilities

- Locked unit

- Chaos during shift change

- Lack of privacy

- Lack of personal space

- A high influx of new admissions requiring acute complex medical care

- Lack of dignity

- Lack of freedom or autonomy

- Lack of structure

To address these factors, take the following steps. (Be sure to include them in your violence-prevention plan.)

- **Create a caring and healing physical environment.** Patients consider a healthcare environment to be healing when they have positive relationships with compassionate caregivers in comfortable and soothing surroundings. A caring-healing environment is one that attends to the patient's body, emotions, mind, and spirit; in which the patient enjoys a therapeutic relationship with caregivers; and in which the patient is actively involved in decisions regarding care (Felgen, 2004).

- **Foster a calm therapeutic environment.** Promote a calm, caring, and healing environment by emphasizing quality, compassionate care. When first meeting patients, introduce yourself and call them by their proper names to show respect in every interaction. Have healthy and respectful interactions with patients, visitors, and interdisciplinary staff, role-modeling respect, courtesy, and kindness in every situation. This fosters an environment of calm, comfort, and caring to promote healing and recovery.

- **Decrease environmental stimulation.** Noise is a particular concern. Decrease noise as much as possible to comfort and calm and foster a healing, recovery-oriented environment.

- **Design the ward for optimal observation.** The best ward design is one in which staff have an unobstructed view of patients in communal areas such as dayrooms, dining rooms, and hallways. Curved Plexiglas mirrors are placed at hallway intersections or concealed areas to maintain safety and visibility. Many facilities have turned to technology, installing closed-circuit video recording cameras in all patient access areas and in high-risk areas such as hallways and providing a dashboard view screen at the nurses' station for safety.

- **Mitigate risks during times of transition.** Staff must be available for therapeutic intervention and de-escalation even during shift changes for safety and continuity of care (Hamrin, Iennaco, & Olsen, 2009).

- **Stagger shifts so they overlap.** This prevents gaps in care during shift changes.

- **Be flexible.** Allow for creative treatment combinations to promote holistic healing and prevent violence.

■ **Reduce agitation during mealtimes.** Patients on mental health units commonly become agitated or even violent during mealtimes. Patients frequently interact during mealtimes, and some of these interactions may turn hostile. There is also the danger of patients pilfering tableware for use later as a weapon. To mitigate this, staff are encouraged to dine with patients. This not only enables staff to monitor patients as well as develop good nurse-patient rapport, but ensures staff are available to de-escalate situations *before* they become out of control or violent.

■ **Promote peer advocates as mentors and facilitators of patient-centered care.** Peer advocates are volunteers who serve as mentors and advisors for patients with mental illness. Peer advocates facilitate collaborative care by acting as patient advisors and intermediaries to promote quality care and optimal recovery outcomes (Henry, Miller-Johnson, Simon, & Schoeny, 2006).

■ **Organize meaningful therapeutic activities.** Include all patients in the unit if possible.

■ **Implement recovery education groups.** Recovery education groups are taught by therapists in mental health facilities to educate and inform patients for holistic, patient-centered care. These could include therapy groups, psycho-education groups, recovery groups, activity groups, exercise groups, conflict-resolution groups, or anger-management groups. These inpatient groups help patients cope with symptoms and navigate the recovery process.

■ **Schedule activities and groups during days, evenings, weekends, and shift changes.** Most mental health facilities provide group therapy Mondays through Fridays, from 8 a.m. to 3 p.m. Very few provide group therapy on evenings or weekends or while staff are in report. Yet research indicates these are the most frequent times of violence and assaults on inpatient mental health units. When there are no groups or activities and boredom takes hold, agitation and violence are often the result (Lanza, Kayne, Hicks, & Milner, 1991). Another dangerous time is during shift report, when the fewest staff members are available on units to monitor patients. Scheduling groups and activities on evenings and weekends as well as during shift report promotes safety, education, and safe holistic care, besides eliminating the dangers of boredom.

- **Post activity schedules.** To provide a predictable structure for patients, mental health inpatient units post a schedule of all daily activities, including mealtimes, vital-signs time, lab-draw times, and group times. In addition, a copy of the schedule is distributed to each patient. This gives patients a sense of structure (Adamson, Vincent, & Cundiff, 2009). Medical units can do the same: provide a schedule that lists times for procedures, tests, and meals to give patients some sense of structure and predictability.

- **Display educational posters around the unit.** Educational posters with bright photos of patients interacting happily with staff on units are an excellent tool to educate patients on appropriate and healthy behavior—particularly for patients on inpatient medical and mental health units. These posters provide a continuous education and learning experience for patients and promote a caring-healing environment.

- **Be consistent.** This applies to staffing and unit organization, rules, the implementation of therapies, and so on.

- **Conduct safety searches upon admission (in mental health facilities).** The idea is to find and remove any contraband or hazardous items for safety. This screening should be performed on all mental health inpatients on their first day in the unit.

- **Decrease or eliminate long lines.** Subjecting inpatients or outpatients to long lines increases their risk of agitation and aggression. Decreasing wait times and long lines eliminates violence triggers and reduces the risk of escalation.

- **Control access to entrances and exits.** Lock unused doors (in accordance with local fire codes) to limit access. This helps control access to patient areas to thwart outsiders intent on doing harm and reduces the risk of physical assault (Gillespie, Gates, Miller, & Howard, 2010).

- **Put on calming music or television programs.** Calming music and television programs can help distract patients and are effective as de-escalation tools to relieve boredom and to soothe agitated patients.

> ✅ **NOTE** Healthcare facilities that offer a calm, safe, therapeutic environment, maintain safe staffing levels, and offer meaningful activities (including group therapy) are likely to experience fewer episodes of violence and to promote optimal recovery outcomes.

- **Foster a predictable, safe, orderly, and respectful environment.** Encourage and facilitate healthy healing interactions with patients in a well-organized, caring, and healing environment. Provide an activity schedule for patients on a mental health unit, or write down a list of care times for patients on a medical unit. This enables you to provide predictable, orderly, respectful, patient-centered care.

- **Minimize sensory deficits.** Provide eyeglasses and hearing aids as needed (Negley & Manley, 1990; Sifford-Snellgrove, Beck, Green, & McSweeney, 2012).

- **Keep environmental stimulation to a minimum.** Lower lights, decrease noise, and promote a calm milieu, or move the agitated patient to another area.

- **Debrief after violent episodes.** This can help you learn techniques to prevent violence from occurring in the future.

ADDRESSING CAREGIVER FACTORS

Caregiver factors can cause an increased risk of aggression. As discussed, these factors include the following. (Note that this list also contains factors relating to interactions between caregivers and patients.)

- Staff educational level
- Lack of training in de-escalation and aggression management
- Staff skills and work experience
- Lack of familiarity with the venue of care
- Lack of familiarity with the patient
- Rigidity of routines
- The physical setting of limits
- Lack of therapeutic communication skills among nurses
- An aloof or uncaring manner
- A lack of emotional and physical availability
- Power struggles
- Nurse overreaction
- Placing too many demands on a patient

Other risk factors pertain to the healthcare provider's personal safety.

Following are several steps to address these factors. (Again, be sure to include these in your violence-prevention plan.)

- **Assess caregiver mental health learning needs.** This will help you identify knowledge gaps for educational and competency development.

- **Provide training in interpersonal skills.** This is effective for preventing violence and improving safety.

- **Boost communication skills.** Providing training in communication skills such as listening, empathy, and role-modeling calmness greatly reduces the risk of patient violence (Rice, Grant, Barney, & Quinsey, 1989).

- **Provide annual training on violence prevention.** One of the best ways to prevent violence is for healthcare staff to obtain education on violence prevention, including physical and verbal techniques. Mental health facility staff are required to attend and participate in Crisis Prevention Institute (CPI) training on an annual basis. This involves training in self-defense, de-escalation, and safety to enable staff to respond appropriately in crisis situations and prevent injuries to staff and patients. It's similar to the Prevention and Management of Disruptive Behavior (PMDB) training program completed by police officers.

> ✓ **NOTE** Educational programs targeting the causes of inpatient violence will greatly improve safety for patients, staff, and everyone else in the healthcare environment.

- **Provide education on maintaining reliability and consistency in therapeutic care.** This improves safety and care outcomes (Chou, Lu, & Mao, 2002; Hamrin et al., 2009; Johnson & Delaney, 2007).

- **Use acuity-based staffing.** Providing adequate staff for observation, monitoring, and early intervention decreases the risk of violence.

- **Intervene early.** Early intervention may prevent further aggression. This is particularly critical when dealing with patients experiencing command hallucinations or delusions.

- **Manage aggressive behavior.** Use assessment techniques and intervention to de-escalate early for safety.

▨ **Offer availability.** Nurses and healthcare staff should tell patients they are available any time to sit down and talk about how they feel. This reduces the risk of violence because the patient will have had an opportunity to talk about issues.

▨ **Knock first and introduce yourself.** When you enter a patient's room, always knock first. Then tell patients who you are, what you are doing, and how long you will be with them. Also explain the steps in each procedure before beginning it.

▨ **Use honorifics.** Call patients by their proper name—for example, Mr. Smith—or simply sir or ma'am.

▨ **Encourage verbalization of issues and precipitating events.** Allowing patients to verbalize their feelings in a nonthreatening environment can help defuse their agitation and possibly prevent future acts of aggression.

▨ **Listen.** Use positive listening. Engage patients. Nod your head to acknowledge that you understand. Repeat back what the patients say to confirm this understanding. Show respect in every interaction.

▨ **Acknowledge and validate the individual's feelings.** If patients are angry, it is OK to say something like, "You seem upset," or "Tell me what you are feeling at this moment." After patients verbalize their issues, it is appropriate to say, "I understand," and "Tell me how I can help you in this situation right now." Make patients aware that you are listening and that you do understand their situation. Finally, offer to help.

▨ **Show respect.** In other words, show consideration or esteem for others. In Western culture, people show respect for each other through the use of honorific terms such as sir or ma'am or by using the person's proper name. Terms of courtesy such as please and thank you also show respect. Research indicates that the primary cause of agitation and violence is when patients feel disrespected (Yonge, 2002; Shaw, 2004; Hamrin et al., 2009; Tingleff, Bradley, Gildberg, Munksgaard, & Hounsgaard, 2017). It is important to show respect quickly when de-escalating the agitated.

▨ **Don't argue, and never shout.** Arguing with patients only intensifies their anger. This drives the escalation cycle and the risk of aggression and violence. Shouting will not make people heard or understood any better. It is also disrespectful and can trigger an aggressive response. Instead, use a professional approach, role-modeling calmness for patients. This may inspire a reciprocal patient response.

- **Model calm.** Taking a calm, matter-of-fact approach not only helps interrupt the cycle of violence, it serves as an example of appropriate behavior for agitated patients.

- **Use nonthreatening body language.** For example, open your hands to expose your palms.

- **Spend more time observing and assessing patients in the therapeutic milieu.** Nurses who spend more time away from the nurses' station interacting with patients on the unit, observing as well as developing nurse-patient therapeutic rapport, encounter less violence. Research indicates nurses who are aloof and do not interact with patients encounter more aggression and violence than nurses who talk to their patients (Lanza et al., 1991).

- **Be reliable and consistent.** Individuals with mental health issues do not trust others easily. When a promise is made, they expect that promise to be kept. Nurses should not promise anything they will not or cannot actually do. If a nurse promises to arrive at a certain time and fails to show up on time, patients may never trust that nurse ever again.

- **Allow patients adequate personal space.** Respect patients' personal boundaries by giving them plenty of room while interacting with them (Sifford-Snellgrove et al., 2012; Umhau, Trandem, Shah, & George, 2012). Also avoid standing within reach of agitated or aggressive patients.

- **Be familiar with safety standards.** This improves both patient safety and staff safety.

- **Minimize personal risk.** Don't tend to agitated patients alone, maintain a clear path to the nearest exit (and leave the door open), wear your hair short or in a bun, avoid wearing clothing or accessories that can be used to injure you (such as earrings that could be pulled or a scarf that could be used to strangle you), know where your colleagues are, and so on (Benveniste, Hibbert, & Runciman, 2005; Boyd, 2008).

PUTTING IT ALL TOGETHER

To help you assemble your own violence-prevention plan, Table 20.1 puts together the various risk factors and solutions discussed in this chapter.

TABLE 20.1 A Sample Violence-Prevention Plan

Risk Factors	Violence Prevention Interventions and Strategies	Rationale
Patient Domain		
Mental instability The presence of delusions The presence of command hallucinations with violent content Poor impulse control Irritability Attention-seeking behavior An agitated state Disorganized thought processes Violation of personal space History of violence Overwhelming stress	**1.** Perform a mental status and risk assessment on admission per facility protocol.	**1.** This helps the nurse and provider identify triggers for aggression and factors that can mitigate or reduce the risk of anger and physical aggression—especially with early intervention.
	2. Intervene and de-escalate early.	**2.** Early intervention and use of de-escalation techniques greatly improves the chances of successful de-escalation to prevent aggression and violence.
	3. Provide patient education (inpatient groups).	**3.** Educating patients helps them develop coping skills and learn systemic and effective approaches to dealing with and mastering tough life situations and problems.
	4. Provide peer mentors for patient support.	**4.** Peer mentors (recovered former patients) provide social support as well as positive role models for recovery.
	5. Provide patient with other outlets for stress and anxiety, such as physical exercise or participation in sports, listening to music, talking to a friend or staff member, or attending support groups.	**5.** Providing an alternative means to channel aggression and angry feelings can help decrease anxiety and stress and help the patient calm down.
	6. Allow for direct communication with caregivers and providers.	**6.** Clear lines of communication establish trust and rapport. Verbalization of feelings may help the patient resolve issues.
	7. Partner with the patient in treatment planning to focus on identifying and meeting individual healthcare needs.	**7.** Patients whose healthcare needs are met are less likely to escalate from tension and stress than patients whose needs go unmet.
	8. Offer PRN (when needed) medication if psychological de-escalation efforts fail and dangerous escalation persists.	**8.** Medications reduce immediate aggression and anxiety to prevent escalation to violence.
	9. Practice one-to-one observation (if called for).	**9.** Patients at high risk for violence require close observation to prevent harm to self or others.
	10. Help the patient identify incentives for optimal behavioral improvement.	**10.** Incentives for behavioral control give patients a goal to reach for as they endeavor to meet the challenges of hospitalization and illness recovery to reduce or prevent the risk of violence.

continues

TABLE 20.1 A Sample Violence-Prevention Plan *(continued)*

Risk Factors	Violence Prevention Interventions and Strategies	Rationale
Patient Domain *(continued)*		
	11. Emphasize the patient's strengths and the hope of recovery.	11. Awareness of strengths promotes hope, which reduces the risks of depression, despondency, and escalation to self-harming behaviors.
Environmental Domain		
Excessive noxious noise Excessive motion Lack of stimulation The ever-changing inpatient population The unpredictable behavior of others Crowded inpatient facilities A locked unit (mental health facilities) Chaos during shift change Lack of privacy Lack of personal space A high influx of new admissions requiring acute and complex medical care Lack of dignity Lack of freedom or autonomy Lack of structure	12. Create a caring and healing physical environment. • Foster a calm therapeutic environment. • Design the ward for optimal observation. • Mitigate risks during times of transition. • Display educational posters around the unit to teach healthy and appropriate behaviors. • Stagger shifts so they overlap to maximize staff availability. • Have staff dine with patients. • Post activity schedules. • Conduct safety searches for contraband or hazardous items (mental health inpatient facilities only). • Decrease or eliminate long lines. • Control access to entrances and exits. • Put on calming music or television programs. • Implement recovery education groups. • Organize meaningful therapeutic activities. • Foster a predictable, safe, orderly, and respectful environment. • Schedule activities and group meetings during days, evenings, weekends, and shift changes.	12. Calm, safe, therapeutic environments that have safe staffing levels and offer meaningful activities and group therapy decrease harmful stimuli and promote optimal recovery outcomes.
	13. Keep environmental stimulation to a minimum.	13. Increased stimulation increases patient anxiety levels, which increases the risk for agitation and aggression.

Risk Factors	Violence Prevention Interventions and Strategies	Rationale
Caregiver Domain		
Staff educational level Lack of training in de-escalation and aggression management Staff skills and work experience Lack of familiarity with the venue of care Lack of familiarity with the patient Rigidity of routines The physical setting of limits Lack of therapeutic communication skills among nurses An aloof or uncaring manner A lack of emotional and physical availability Power struggles Nurse overreaction Placing too many demands on a patient Compromising the safety of the healthcare provider	**14.** Perform a mental health learning needs assessment on caregivers to identify gaps for educational and competency development in the following areas: • De-escalation training • Violence-prevention training • Crisis-intervention training • Management of aggressive behavior • Conflict-resolution training • CPI or PMDB training • Therapeutic communication training • Interpersonal skill development • Early intervention and de-escalation	**14.** Education and training in early therapeutic intervention, risks, communication skills, and de-escalation and violence-prevention techniques reduce the risk of encountering violence.
	15. Offer availability to talk and encourage verbalization of issues and precipitating events.	**15.** Verbalization of feelings in a non-threatening environment can defuse agitation.
	16. Engage in therapeutic communication by doing the following: • Introduce yourself. • Call the patient by the proper name (e.g., Mr. or Mrs. Smith, or sir or ma'am). • Use active listening. • Acknowledge and validate the person's feelings. • Encourage patients to discuss their feelings. • Show respect in your words and interactions.	**16.** Developing therapeutic rapport and showing respect reduces the risk of aggression.
	17. Remain calm and nonconfrontational. Do the following: • Don't argue and never shout. • Model calmness. • Use nonthreatening body language.	**17.** Taking a calm, matter-of-fact approach can help interrupt the cycle of violence.

continues

TABLE 20.1 A Sample Violence-Prevention Plan *(continued)*

Risk Factors	Violence Prevention Interventions and Strategies	Rationale
Caregiver Domain *(continued)*		
	18. Debrief.	**18.** Discussing events can lead to better understanding and decrease emotional impact as well as preventing possible future violent or aggressive acts.
	19. Spend time observing and assessing patients in the therapeutic milieu.	**19.** Early intervention may prevent aggressive responses to command hallucinations or delusions.
	20. Be reliable and consistent.	**20.** This is essential for developing trust and therapeutic rapport.
	21. Allow patients adequate personal space and minimize personal risk. For example, keep doors open, wear short hair and post earrings (rather than ones that dangle), and avoid wearing objects around your neck.	**21.** Know the unit's safety precautions for staff and patients inside and out to prevent injury.
	22. Use acuity-based staffing.	**22.** Providing adequate staff for observation, monitoring, and early intervention with de-escalation decreases the risk of violence.

IN CONCLUSION

The healthcare violence-prevention plan in Table 20.1 recognizes the critical origins of violence and provides effective strategies to prevent violence in healthcare facilities for safe holistic care. A healthcare violence-prevention plan and de-escalation educational program that addresses the holistic risk factor domains of patient, environment, and caregiver are very effective methods to reduce or even prevent healthcare violence. The healthcare violence-prevention plan suggested is a comprehensive therapeutic program that educates and implements best practices in violence prevention and promotes a safe healthcare environment.

Healthcare violence is preventable with early assessment and intervention using de-escalation strategies for safety. Having an organized healthcare violence-prevention plan and de-escalation educational program that targets the causes of inpatient violence will greatly improve safety for patients, staff, and everyone else in the healthcare environment. Safety is improved with the holistic application of interventions that focus on patient, caregiver, and environmental risk factors to prevent violence. The holistic application of de-escalation techniques to prevent violence offers immense benefits for healthcare staff and the workplace environment. It is truly the future of safe healthcare practice—providing safety; improving the lives of our vulnerable patient populations; and promoting health, wellness, and recovery.

REFERENCES

Adamson, M. A., Vincent, A. A., & Cundiff, J. (2009).Common ground not a battle ground. Violence prevention at a detoxification facility. *Journal of Psychosocial Nursing and Mental Health Services, 47*(8), 28–35. doi: 10.3928/02793695-20090706-01

American Psychiatric Association, American Psychiatric Nurses Association, & National Association of Psychiatric Health Systems. (2007). *Learning from each other: Success stories and ideas for reducing restraint/seclusion in behavioral health.* Retrieved from http://www.restraintfreeworld.org/documents/Learning%20From%20Each%20Other.pdf

Benveniste, K., Hibbert, P., & Runciman, W. (2005). Violence in health care: The contribution of the Australian Patient Safety Foundation to incident monitoring and analysis. *Medical Journal of Australia, 183*(7), 348–351.

Boyd, M. A. (2008). *Psychiatric nursing: Contemporary practice* (4th ed.). Philadelphia, PA: Lippincott, Williams & Wilkins.

Chou, K. R., Lu, R. B., & Mao, W. C. (2002). Factors relevant to patient assaultive behavior and assault in acute inpatient psychiatric units in Taiwan. *Archives of Psychiatric Nursing, 16*(4), 187–195.

Felgen, J. (2004). A caring and healing environment. *Nursing Administration Quarterly, 28*(4), 288–301. doi: 10.1097/00006216-200410000-00012

Gillespie, G. L., Gates, D. M., Miller, M., & Howard, P. K. (2010). Workplace violence in healthcare settings: Risk factors and protective strategies. *Rehabilitation Nursing, 35*(5), 177–184.

Hamrin, V., Iennaco, J., & Olsen, D. (2009). A review of ecological factors affecting inpatient psychiatric unit violence: Implications for relational and unit cultural improvements. *Issues in Mental Health Nursing, 30*(4), 214–226. doi: 10.1080/01612840802701083

Henry, D. B., Miller-Johnson, S., Simon, T. R., & Schoeny, M. E. (2006). Validity of teacher ratings in selecting influential aggressive adolescents for a targeted preventive intervention. *Prevention Science, 7*(1), 31–41.

Hodgins, S. (2008). Violent behaviour among people with schizophrenia: A framework for investigations of causes, and effective treatment, and prevention. *Philosophical Transactions of the Royal Society of London, Series B, Biological Sciences, 363*(1503), 2,505–2,518. doi: 10.1098/rstb.2008.0034

Johnson, M. E., & Delaney, K. R. (2007). Keeping the unit safe: The anatomy of escalation. *Journal of the American Psychiatric Nurses Association, 13*(1), 42–50.

Lanza, M. L., Kayne, H. L., Hicks, C., & Milner, J. (1991). Nursing staff characteristics related to patient assault. *Issues in Mental Health Nursing, 12*(3), 253–265.

Negley, E. N. & Manley, J. T. (1990). Environmental interventions in assaultive behavior. *Journal of Gerontological Nursing, 16*(3), 29–33.

Rice, M., Grant, T., Barney, G., & Quinsey, V. (1989). *Violence in institutions, prediction and control.* Toronto, ON: Hogrete and Huber Publishers.

Shaw, M. M. (2004). Aggression toward staff by nursing home residents: Findings from a grounded theory study. *Journal of Gerontological Nursing, 30*(10), 43–54.

Sifford-Snellgrove, S. K., Beck, C., Green, A., & McSweeney, J. C. (2012). Victim or initiator? Certified nursing assistants' perceptions of resident characteristics that contribute to resident-to-resident violence in nursing homes. *Research in Gerontological Nursing, 5*(1), 55–63. doi: 10.3928/19404921-20110603-01

Tingleff, E. B., Bradley, S. K., Gildberg, F. A., Munksgaard, G., & Hounsgaard, L. (2017). "Treat me with respect." A systematic review and thematic analysis of psychiatric patients' reported perceptions of the situations associated with the process of coercion. *Journal of Psychiatric and Mental Health Nursing, 24*(9), 681–698. doi: 10.1111/jpm.12410

Umhau, J. C., Trandem, K., Shah, M., & George, D. T. (2012). The physician's unique role in preventing violence: A neglected opportunity? *BMC Medicine, 10*, 146. doi: 10.1186/1741-7015-10-146

Yonge, O. (2002). Psychiatric patients' perceptions of constant care. *Journal of Psychosocial Nursing and Mental Health Services, 40*(6), 22–29.

INDEX

> ✔ **NOTE** An *f* in page references is for figures; a *t* in page references is for tables.

A

Academy of Child & Adolescent Psychiatry (AACAP), 235
accidents, stress and, 78
accommodating, 96*f,* 97
accountability, 54
activation phase, 34
activities
    group, 253
    schedules, 254
acute stress, 79
admissions
    influx of, 17
    risk assessments, 142, 143*f*
advice, avoiding giving, 68
advocates, peer, 253
affect, evaluating, 130–131
aggression
    assessment of aggressive situations, 6
    definition of, 14
    mental health emergencies, 114
    pathways for, 2–4
    pharmacological interventions, 3
    phases of, 30
    physical interventions, 3–4
    prevention, 7–8
    psychological interventions, 2–3
    responses to, 3
    risk of, 248–249
    stress management (*see* stress management)
    triggers, 36–38
    variables and risk factors for, 13–27
aggressive phase, 33*t*
agitated phase, 33*t*
agitation
    assessment, 41–42
    communication, 62 (*see also* therapeutic communication)
    de-escalation (*see* de-escalation)
    dementia and, 183
    distractions, 48–49
    during mealtimes, 253
alcohol, 115
    abuse, 115
    mental health emergencies, 114
    withdrawal patients, 121
Alcoholics Anonymous (AA), 120
alertness, evaluating, 129–131
alert to safety, 8
algorithms, de-escalation, 33*t*
alliances, developing, 107
Alzheimer's disease, 22, 49, 182
American Psychiatric Association (APA), 2, 126, 170, 235
American Psychiatric Nurses Association (APNA), 2

anger, 41. *See also* angry patients
    expressions of, 214–215, 218
    management, 47, 218, 221t
    origins of, 216–217
    patterns of, 217
    progressive muscular relaxation
      (PMR), 219
    reorienting to reality, 50–51
    schizophrenia, 152
    stress management (*see* stress
      management)
    triggers, 216–217
    verbalizing, 47
angry patients
    anger management, 221t
    assessments, 217–218
    communications, 220
    de-escalation, 213–222
    definition of, 214
    expressions of anger, 214–215
    origins of anger, 216–217
    preventing escalation, 218–220
annual training, 256
anticipated life crises, 106
anxiety, 23, 159–163. *See also* panic disorder
    dementia and, 183
    mental health emergencies, 114
    patients, 250
    progressive muscular relaxation
      (PMR), 219
    releasing, 47
    reorienting to reality, 50–51
    verbalizing, 47
anxious phase, 33t
appropriateness, 64
arguments, 48, 257
aromatherapy, 187
assault cycle, 6, 34–36, 34t–35t
assaultive behavior, 16
assessments
    aggressive situations, 6
    angry patients, 217–218
    assault cycle, 34–36
    bipolar disorder, 154–157

delirium, 195–196
dementia, 182–184
difficult patients, 206–207
escalating situations, 29–44
escalation cycles, 30–33
legal status, 128
major depressive disorder, 154–157
mental health, 5–6, 116–118, 256 (*see also*
    mental health)
mental status, 125–147
motor activity, 135–137
non-suicidal self-injury (NSSI), 173–174
panic disorder, 159–163
physical appearance, 128
risk, 137–143
schizophrenia, 150–151
signs of agitation, 41–42
speech, 135–137
thought processes, 132–133
verbal techniques for de-escalation,
    46–47
violent patients, 142
attention-seeking behavior, 129
attitudes
    evaluating, 129–131
    maintaining professional, 67
    types of, 130t
audience, removing, 52
auditory hallucinations, 150
authenticity, 65
autonomy, lack of, 18
availability, 257
awareness of surroundings, 225

B

baby boomers, stress and, 81
badges, being aware of, 227
balance, 47
behavioral theory, 216
behaviors
    accountability for, 54
    aggression, 3 (*see also* aggression)
    anger, 214–215 (*see also* angry patients)
    assaultive, 16

calming techniques (*see* calming
    techniques)
caring, 243
correct, 209
criminal, 16
crisis state, 105
difficult patients, 204
escalation, 39–40, 56
evaluating, 129–131
incorrect, 209
management, 256
mental health emergencies, 114
non-suicidal self-injury (NSSI), 170*t*
predictability of, 17
proactive, 8
staff-splitting, 204
biologic theory, 216
bipolar disorder, 21, 51, 150, 154–157
    comparing mental disorders and,
        163*t*–165*t*
    definition of, 154
    symptoms, 155*t*
biting, 171. *See also* non-suicidal self-injury
    (NSSI)
body language, 53, 62, 63*f*, 225–227, 258
borderline personality disorder, 23, 162
brain injuries, 22
breathing exercises, 83. *See also* holistic stress
    management
buddy systems, 153, 228–231
bullying, cyber-bullying, 171
burning, 170. *See also* non-suicidal self-injury
    (NSSI)

C

CAGE (cut down, annoyed, guilty,
    eye-opener), 120
calming techniques, 97, 252, 254, 258
    bipolar disorder patients, 156
    comfort measures, 49–50
    delirium, 197
    healthcare environments, 239–246
    remaining calm, 52

verbal techniques for de-escalation,
    46–47
cancer, stress and, 78
caregivers
    communications with, 250
    online resources for, 11
    risks, 6
    variables for aggression, 18–20
    violence-prevention plans, 255–258
    working with, 9–11
caring
    behaviors, 243
    environments, 239–246
    theories, 243–245
    universal culture, 245
case studies
    anger management, 221
    buddy systems, 230–231
    dementia, 189
    mental health emergencies, 122–123
    risk assessments, 145
catastrophizing, 218
chaos, 17, 50
chemical restraints, 3
choices, offering, 54
chronic depression, 206
chronic stress, 79
cirrhosis of the liver, stress and, 78
clarifying, 66
Cocaine Anonymous (CA), 120
cognition, 194
collaboration, 96, 96*f*
    patients, 143
    treatments, 250
collegial relationships, building, 242
combative behavior, 129
comfort measures, 49–50, 187
communications, 37, 40. *See also* behaviors
    about medical procedures, 185
    angry patients, 220
    with caregivers, 250
    concise, 53
    conflict resolution, 98
    crisis intervention, 109–110

de-escalation, 46 (*see also* de-escalation)
delirium, 199
difficult patients, 208–210
with difficult patients, 208
open communication rules, 99
skills, 256
tailoring, 67
therapeutic for de-escalation, 60–73
Therapeutic Interdisciplinary Team
    Communication, 238
compassion, 241
competing, 96, 96f
compromising, 96, 96f
concise communication, 53
confidentiality, 67
conflicts
    benefits of conflict resolution, 94–95
    definition of, 94
    elements of conflict resolution, 97–99
    open communication rules, 99
    resolution, 5, 93–101
    styles of conflict resolution, 95–97
    types of, 95
confusion, 37
congruence, 65
consistency, 54, 254, 256, 258
coping skills, 197
coronary heart disease (CHD), stress and, 78
correct behavior, 209
covert conflict, 95
criminal behavior, 16
crisis intervention, 103–111
    behaviors, 105
    communication, 109–110
    crisis reflecting psychopathology, 106
    definition of crisis, 104
    phases of, 107–109
    stages of crisis development, 104
    types of crises, 106–107
crisis intervention teams (CITs), 228
crisis phase, 6, 31, 34
crisis prevention intervention (CPI), 228
Culture Care Diversity and Universality
    Theory, 245

cutting, 170. *See also* non-suicidal self-injury
    (NSSI)
cyber-bullying, 171
cycles
    assault, 34–36, 34t–35t
    of emotions, 31
    escalation, 30–33, 31f, 33t
    therapeutic communication, 60–61f

D

debriefing, 8–9, 255
debriefing patients/staffs, 234–236
deep breathing, 219
de-escalation
    algorithms, 33t
    angry patients, 213–222
    definition of, 46
    delirium, 193–202
    dementia, 181–191
    distractions for, 48–49
    for holistic wellness, 1–12
    incident processes (*see* incidents)
    interventions, 143
    milieu management, 51–52
    non-suicidal self-injury (NSSI), 169–179
    overview of, 2
    pathways for aggression, 2–4
    of patients with mental disorders,
        149–167
    plans, 143–144, 144f
    principles of, 52–56
    processes, 5–10
    reorienting to reality, 50–51
    response tools, 4–5
    safety during, 223–232
    techniques, 7–8, 32, 45–58
    therapeutic communication for, 60–73
    verbal techniques for, 46–48
    violence-prevention plans, 247–264
delirium, 22, 193–202
    assessments, 195–196
    communications, 199
    definition of, 194

medical conditions associated with, 195*t*
origins of, 195
preventing escalation, 196–198
safety of patients with, 201
working with family members, 200–201
delusions, 134–135, 142
    schizophrenia, 150
    types of, 135
dementia, 22, 49, 51, 181–191
    assessments, 182–184
    case studies, 189
    definition of, 182
    guidelines for care, 186
    preventing escalation, 184–186
    quality of life, 189–190
dependent behavior, 129
depression, 23
    chronic depression, 206
    dementia and, 183
    holistic wellness, 77
    reducing symptoms of, 60
    stress management (*see* stress management)
detoxification, 119
developmental crises, 106
Diagnostic and Statistical Manual of Mental Disorders (DSM-5)
    delirium, 194
    non-suicidal self-injury (NSSI), 170
    panic attacks, 160
diaphragmatic breathing, 83–84
difficult patients
    assessments, 206–207
    characteristics of, 205*t*
    communications, 208–210
    de-escalation of, 204–212
    definition of, 204
    elderly patients, 211–212
    origins of behaviors, 205–206
    preventing escalation, 207–208
dignity, lack of, 117
dispositional crises, 106
distractions for de-escalation, 48–49
distress, 79

diversional activities, 49
documentation, 8–9, 236–238
domestic violence, 115
drug abuse, 115
dysfunction in families, 10

E

early intervention, 29–44, 256
education, 18
    annual training, 256
    patients, 249
    posters, 254
    recovery phase, 253
efficiency, 64
elderly patients as difficult patients, 211–212
electroconvulsive therapy (ECT), 151
emergencies
    managing mental health, 113–124
    psychiatric, 107
    response codes, 3
emotional availability, 19
emotions, 77
    anger, 41
    cycles of, 31
    lowering tension, 46 (*see also* de-escalation)
    validating, 257
empathy, 65, 241
entrances, controlling, 254
environments
    variables for aggression, 16–18
    violence-prevention plans, 251–255
escalation
    angry patients, 218–220
    behaviors, 39–40, 56
    cycles, 30–33, 31*f,* 33*t*
    delirium, 196–198
    difficult patients, 207–208
    phase, 31
    phases, 6, 34
    preventing, 184–186
    risks of, 8
    situation assessments, 29–44

eustress, 79
evaluating conflict resolution, 98
exclusive meditation, 87
exercise, 50–51, 219
exits, controlling, 254
expression, methods of, 37

F

face-to-face communication, 61
facial expressions, 62
facilities, crowding of, 17
families
    online resources for, 11
    working with, 9–11
fears, verbalizing, 47
feedback, 64, 65f, 66, 212
firearms, 119
flashbacks, 105
flexibility, 64
focusing, 66–67, 98
follow-through, 55
freedom, lack of, 18
Freud, Sigmund, 47
frustration, 37, 183
fundamental human elements, 76–78

G

gathering information about crises, 108
Generation Xers, stress and, 81
genuineness, 65
gestures, 62
goals of difficult patients, 208–209
grief, managing, 188
groups
    activities, 253
    communication, 64
guided mental imagery, 84–87

H

hair, and accessories, 227
hallucinations, 105, 134–135, 150, 152

healing
    healthcare environments, 239–246
    relationships, 241
    therapeutic communication, 60
    treatment environments, 8
healthcare environments
    conflicts, 94
    healing, 239–246
    stress in, 76
Health Insurance Portability and
  Accountability Act (HIPAA) of 1996, 128
history of violence, 16
holistic stress management, 81–83. *See also*
  stress management
    diaphragmatic breathing, 83–84
    meditation, 87–88
    mental imagery, 84–87
    progressive muscular relaxation (PMR),
      88–90
holistic wellness, 77f
homicidal ideation, 141, 152
honorifics, 257

I

impulsivity, 134
incentives for improvement, 251
incidents
    debriefing patients/staffs, 234–236
    processes after, 233–238
    reporting, 236–238
inclusive meditation, 87
incorrect behavior, 209
independence, 196
infections, 22
information, repeating, 211
inpatient populations, 17
insight, 134
intellect, 77
interactions, variables for aggression, 20
interpersonal communication, 63, 256
intervention
    allowing patients to choose, 54
    anger management, 221t

bipolar disorder patients, 155 (*see also* bipolar disorder)

conflict resolution, 99

crisis, 103–111 (*see also* crisis intervention)

crisis prevention intervention (CPI), 228

de-escalation, 143 (*see* de-escalation)

early, 29–44, 256

importance of, 42

mental health emergencies, 114

panic attacks, 161–162

pathways for aggression, 2–4

staying safe during, 223–232

interviews, 116, 126. *See also* assessments

intrapersonal communication, 64

intrusive thoughts, 105

isolative behavior, 130

isometric exercises, 187

J

jewelry, being aware of, 227

Joint Commission (JC), 2, 4, 9, 126, 138, 143

debriefing requirements, 236

reporting, 237

judgment, 55, 68, 134

Jung, Carl, 76

L

learning theory (NSSI), 173

legal status assessments, 128

Leininger, Madeline, 245

Lewin's change model, 219–220

lighting, effect on patients, 52

limits, setting, 53–54, 209

listening, 66, 257

to bipolar disorder patients, 156

conflict resolution, 98

locked units, 17

loops, feedback, 65*f*

lung ailments, stress and, 78

M

major depressive disorder, 150, 157–159

comparing mental disorders and, 163*t*–165*t*

definition of, 157

symptoms, 158*t*

management

anger, 218, 221*t* (*see also* anger)

assault cycles, 34*t*–35*t*

behaviors, 256

grief, 188

mental health emergencies, 113–124

milieu, 51–52

stress management, 75–92

mantras, 87

Marijuana Anonymous (MA), 120

massages, 49

maturational crises, 106

meals, 17, 50

medical records, 117, 162

medications

bipolar disorder, 156

panic attacks, 162

schizophrenia, 153

meditation, 87–88, 219

memory status, 133, 197–198

mental disorders, 23

bipolar disorder, 154–157

borderline personality disorder, 23, 162

comparing conditions, 163–165

de-escalation of patients with, 149–167

major depressive disorder, 157–159

panic disorder, 159–163

schizophrenia, 150–154

mental health

aiding suicidal patients, 118–119

assessments, 5–6, 116–118, 256

definition of emergencies, 114

managing emergencies, 113–124

substance abuse patients, 119–121

types of emergencies, 115

violent patients, 121–123

mental imagery, 84–87, 219
mental status assessments, 125–147
    de-escalation plans, 143–144, 144*f*
    delusions, 134–135
    evaluations, 129–131
    hallucinations, 134–135
    insight, 134
    intellect, 134
    judgment, 134
    legal status, 128
    motor activity, 135–137
    physical appearance, 128
    risk assessments, 137–143
    speech, 135–137
    templates, 127*f*
    thought processes, 132–133
mentors, peer, 250
milieu management, 51–52
millennials, stress and, 81
misunderstandings, 38
Model of Human Care, 243–244
monitoring, one-to-one, 8
moods, 131
    evaluating, 129–131
    mental health emergencies, 114
motion, 16
motivation, decreased, 129
motor activity assessments, 135–137
multisensory stimulation, 187
music, listening to, 51, 162, 199

N

Narcotics Anonymous (NA), 120
National Association of Psychiatric Health
   Systems (NAPHS), 2, 235
National Institute for Occupational Safety
   and Health (NIOSH), 2
negative expressions of anger, 214–215
negative self-talk, 214
negotiations, conflict resolution, 98
neurocognitive disorders, 182
neustress, 79
nightmares, 105

noises as triggers, 51
non-suicidal self-injury (NSSI), 169–179
    assessments, 173–174
    behaviors, 170*t*
    definition of, 170
    differentiating from suicidal ideation,
       176–177, 177*t*
    origins of behavior, 171–173
    prevention, 174–175
    reversing, 176
nonthreatening language, 68
nonverbal communication, 61–63, 65
noxious noise, 16

O

objective professional approaches (to conflict
   resolution), 97
observation, 258
    one-to-one, 251
    optimizing, 252
observations, 126. *See also* assessments
one-to-one monitoring, 8
one-to-one observation, 251
online resources for caregivers/families, 11
open communication rules, 99
open-ended questions, 47
opening-up meditation, 87
organic brain syndrome (OBS), 22
organic disorders, 22
orientation, evaluating, 129–131
overstimulation, 51
overt conflict, 95

P

pain, 38
panic attacks, 160
panic disorder, 150, 159–163
    comparing mental disorders and,
       163*t*–165*t*
    definition of, 160
    levels of, 159–160
    symptoms of panic attacks, 160*t*
paraverbals, 53, 67

pathways for aggression, 2–4
    pharmacological interventions, 3
    physical interventions, 3–4
    psychological interventions, 2–3
patients
    aiding violent, 121–123
    alcohol withdrawal, 121
    angry (*see* angry patients)
    anxiety, 250
    with bipolar disorder, 154–157
    buddy systems, 228–231
    collaboration, 143
    debriefing, 234–236
    de-escalation of with mental disorders,
      149–167
    with delirium, 193–202
    with dementia, 181–191
    difficult (*see* difficult patients)
    education, 249
    lack of familiarity with, 19
    with major depressive disorder, 157–159
    managing grief, 188
    non-suicidal self-injury (NSSI), 169–179
    with panic disorder, 159–163
    personal space, 225, 258
    reorienting to reality, 50–51
    safety, 116, 153, 224
    saving face, 53
    with schizophrenia, 150–154
    stress, 250
    threatening, 228
    types of difficult, 204
    variables for aggression, 15–16
    violence-prevention plans, 248–251
    working with family members, 9–11
patterns of anger, 217
peer advocates, 253
peer mentors, 250
perceptions, 218
personality disorders, 206
personal space, 17, 37, 225, 258
person-to-person interviews, 126
pet therapy, 186
pharmacological interventions, 3

phases
    activation, 34
    of aggression, 30
    aggressive, 33*t*
    agitated, 33*t*
    anxious, 33*t*
    crisis, 31, 34
    of crisis intervention, 107–109
    escalation, 31, 33*t* , 34
    post-crisis depression, 34–35
    recovery, 34–35
    stabilization, 34, 36
    trigger, 30
    violence, 33*t*
physical appearance, 128
physical availability, 19
physical bodies, 77
physical disability, 38
physical environments, creating caring,
    240–241, 252
physical interventions, 3–4
physical limitations, 19
plans, violence-prevention, 247–264
poisoning, 119
positive expressions of anger, 214–215
positive reinforcement, 55
post-crisis depression phase, 34–35
posture, 62
pranayama, 83
preventing escalation
    aggression, 7–8
    angry patients, 218–220
    difficult patients, 207–208
    non-suicidal self-injury (NSSI), 174–175
    violence, 2, 126–127
    violence-prevention plans, 247–264
principles of de-escalation, 52–56
privacy, lack of, 17
proactive behavior, 8
problem-solving, 5, 67, 109
processes
    after incidents, 233–238
    debriefing patients/staffs, 234–236
    de-escalation, 5–10
    reporting, 236–238

progression of escalating behaviors, 40f
progressive muscular relaxation (PMR), 88–90, 219
protocols, safety, 224
proxemics, 62
psychiatric emergencies, 107
psychiatric triage, reasons for seeking, 114, 115
psychoanalytic theory, 216
psychological de-escalation techniques, 46. *See also* de-escalation
psychological interventions, 2–4
psychopharmacology, 150
psychosis, 23
psychosocial treatments, 151
psychotic disorders, 114, 206

Q

questions
    open-ended, 47
    questioning patients, 68

R

rage, 215. *See also* anger
rapport, 107, 118
rationality, 67
reality
    combining with theories, 67
    presenting, 66
    reorienting to, 153
recovery phase, 34–35, 250, 253
redirections, 153
relationships, healing, 241
relaxation exercises, 50–51, 62
relaxation recordings, 187
reliability, 256, 258
reminiscence therapy, 49, 188
reorienting to reality, 50–51
repetitive behavior, 130
reporting, 8–9, 236–238
resolutions
    conflicts, 5
    promoting, 47

respect, 36, 53, 65, 257
responses
    to stress, 78–79
    tools, 4–5
restraints, chemical, 3
restrictive meditation, 87
reversing non-suicidal self-injury (NSSI), 176
risks, 13–27
    admissions, 142
    of aggression, 248–249
    assessments, 137–143
    case studies, 145
    conditions associated with, 24f
    of escalation, 8
    escalation behaviors, 40
    minimizing personal, 258
    to patients, 6
    patient variables for, 15–16
    procedures, 138f
    screening aggression, 7
    of stress, 76
    during transitions, 252
ritualistic behavior, 129
role models, anger, 218
role playing, 212
routines, 19
Ruesch, Jurgen, 60

S

safety
    aiding suicidal patients, 118–119
    awareness of surroundings, 225
    body language, 225–227
    buddy systems, 228–231
    during de-escalation, 223–232
    hair, and accessories, 227
    implementing, 7
    patients, 116, 153, 224
    of patients with delirium, 201
    personal space, 225
    protocols, 224
    safety first, 32
    searches, 254
    standards, 258

saving face, 53
schedules
    activities, 254
    for delirium patients, 197
schizoid conditions, 206
schizophrenia, 21, 150–154
    comparing mental disorders and,
        163t–165t
    definition of, 150
    treatment of, 150–151
schizotypal conditions, 206
self-awareness, 62, 66
self-care, 76, 196
self-control, 30f, 47
self-destructive behaviors, 214–215. *See also*
    angry patients
self-disclosure, 67
self-esteem, 37–38
self-injuries, 171. *See also* non-suicidal
    self-injury (NSSI)
self-talk, 214
sense of purpose, 37
sensory deficits, 255
sharing de-escalation duties, 55
shift changes, 17
shouting, avoiding, 257
signs of agitation, 41–42
silence, 66
Simonton, Carl, 84
Simonton, Stephanie, 84
skills, 18
    anger management, 47
    communications, 256
    coping, 197
    crisis intervention, 104 (*see also* crisis
        intervention)
    interpersonal communication, 256
    psychological de-escalation
        techniques, 46 (*see also* de-escalation)
    therapeutic communication, 19
societal communication, 64
sociocultural theory, 216
speech
    assessments, 135–137
    slowing down, 211

spirit, 77
spoken-word communication, 61
stabilization phase, 34, 36
staffs
    caring healthcare environments,
        241–242
    debriefing, 234–236
staff-splitting behavior, 129, 204
stages of crisis development, 104
standards, safety, 258
statistics, violence, 16
stimulation, 16, 252
stress. *See also* stress management
    acute, 79
    chronic, 79
    crises (*see* crisis intervention)
    delirium, 197
    patients, 250
    reducing, 50–51
stress management, 75–92
    causes of stress, 80–81
    fundamental human elements, 76–78
    holistic stress management, 81–83
    stress responses, 78–79
    types of stress, 79–80
structure, lack of, 18
substance abuse, 16, 22, 115
    aiding patients, 119–121
    mental health emergencies, 114
suffocation, 119
suicide, 114–115
    aiding suicidal patients, 118–119
    assessments, 116–117
    differentiating non-suicidal self-injury
        (NSSI) from, 176–177, 177t
    holistic wellness, 77
    major depressive disorder, 158
    methods of, 118–119
    risk assessment, 138
    stress and, 78
    stress management (*see* stress
        management)
    templates for assessments, 139f
summarizing, 66

suspicions, dementia and, 183
symptoms
    of bipolar disorder, 155t
    of major depressive disorder, 158t
    of panic attacks, 160t

T

takedowns, 3
tattoos, 171
teams, 228. See also buddy systems
    sharing de-escalation duties, 55
    team efforts, 55
    Therapeutic Interdisciplinary Team
        Communication, 238
templates
    admission risk assessments, 143f
    homicidal ideation, 141f
    mental status assessments, 127f
    suicide assessments, 139f
tension
    lowering, 46
    progressive muscular relaxation
        (PMR), 219
    releasing, 47
theories
    behavioral, 216
    biologic, 216
    caring, 243–245
    combining with reality, 67
    Culture Care Diversity and Universality
        Theory, 245
    Model of Human Care, 243–244
    psychoanalytic, 216
    sociocultural, 216
therapeutic activities, 253
therapeutic communication
    contexts, 63–64
    criteria for successful, 64–65
    cycles, 60–61, 61f
    for de-escalation, 60–73
    definition of, 60
    elements of, 65–66
    goals of, 60

with the hard-of-hearing, 68–69
nonverbal communication, 61–63
skills, 19
techniques, 66–69
trust, 69–71
verbal communication, 61–63
therapeutic milieu, 51
therapy
    pet, 186
    reminiscence, 49, 188
thought content, 133t
thought processes, assessments, 132–133
thought-stopping, 153
threatening patients, 228
tools, response, 4–5
training, 18, 256. See also education
transitions, risks during, 252
traumatic crises, 106
treatments
    collaboration, 250
    for panic disorder, 162
    schizophrenia, 150–151
triggers
    aggression, 36–38
    anger, 216–217
    phase, 6, 30, 139
    violence, 36–38
trust, 65, 69–71, 107, 118

U

universal culture caring, 245

V

validating emotions, 257
variables for aggression, 13–27
    caregivers, 18–20
    environmental, 16–18
    interactions, 20
    patients, 15–16
ventilation, 47
venues of care, familiarity of, 18–19
verbal communication, 61–63, 65

verbalization, 162, 257
    difficult patients and, 208
    encouraging, 60
verbal techniques for de-escalation, 46–48
violence
    accountability for, 54
    aiding violent patients, 121–123
    assessments, 142
    definition of, 14
    history of, 16
    ideation, 141
    origins of, 14
    phase, 33*t*
    prevention of, 2, 126–127
    rage, 215
    risk for harmful intent, 15
    statistics, 16
    stress management (*see* stress
      management)
    triggers, 36–38

violence-prevention plans, 247–264
    caregivers, 255–258
    environmental factors, 251–255
    patient factors, 248–251
    sample of, 259*t*–262*t*
visual airs, 211
visualization techniques, 162
vocational counseling, 151

W

walking, 50
warning signs of dementia, 182–183
Watson, Jean, 243–244
weapons, access to, 15
withdrawn behavior, 130
work experience, 18
written communication, 61

Y

yoga, 83